Praise for

AGELESS, PAINLESS TENNIS

"A must read for weekend warriors and advanced athletes alike looking to heal nagging injuries and prevent future ones!"

> **—Brad Gilbert**, Former World #4, Coach, ESPN Tennis Analyst, Author of *Winning Ugly*

"David Smith has pulled off a form of magic. In a radical act of alchemy, he has turned simple and effective movements into improved tennis performance. Believe it or not, solving musculoskeletal pain is actually the low bar. Don't be fooled. David is more interested in you playing savage tennis for the rest of your life. This book is a gift that will keep on giving."

> **—Dr. Kelly Starrett,** DPT, Coach, *New York Times* Best-Selling Author of *Becoming a Supple Leopard* and *Ready to Run: Unlocking Your Potential to Run Naturally*

"David has masterfully captured cutting-edge principles to achieve physical and mental wellness that will keep you pain-free and active for a lifetime."

> **—Jeff Greenwald**, MFT., Author of *The Best Tennis of Your Life* and Two-Time World Champion

"The leader in the clubhouse out of all the athletic books I've read in this area. David is the real deal and knows this stuff inside out. A must read for all parents, coaches and players!!!

> **—Rick Macci**, World-Renowned Coach, Uspta Hall of Fame

"Read this book if you want to avoid injury. David's simple tips will keep you healthy and happy on the tennis courts for many years to come."

—**Peter Wright**, UC Berkeley Men's Tennis Coach, Former Irish Davis Cup Captain

"*Ageless Painless Tennis* by David Starbuck Smith will make you feel like a kid again. Get ready to enjoy tennis for the rest of your life! I now look forward to coaching and playing into my 90s."

—**Angel Lopez**, Director of Tennis San Diego Tennis and Racquet Club, 1999 United States Olympic Committee/USTA Development Coach of the Year, 1995 USPTA National Professional of the Year, 2005 Professional Tennis Registry International Professional of the Year

"After dealing with rotator cuff tendinitis for ten years, it only took about six weeks of doing the exercises to fully heal my shoulder and completely relieve the pain. From that my serve speed has increased and overall my body feels strong and pain-free which ultimately helps me feel better and perform better on the court."

—**Maria Sanchez**, WTA #51 Ranked Doubles Player in the World

"Today, I am 60 years young, my doubles partner and I won the 2019 National Championships in Arizona for the 50+. We beat seven teams from around the country, and not once did I feel pain, and yes, I do the pre-tennis routine and post-tennis routine before and after every match. I highly recommend this book, it will change your life. Thank you, David."

—**Marty Briesach**, 4.5+ 2019 National 50s Doubles Champion

"In my personal crusade to just manage the pain of decades of back spasms and disk issues, I stumbled upon David Smith—I no longer have to manage pain. David eliminated it. David is singularly the best body mechanic I've ever met and I've tried everything, as you might imagine. I have done David's routines for years now and play tennis with reckless abandon, knowing my body is balanced and can take it. He is a truly gifted individual."

—J. Michael Tierney, USTA 4.5

Ageless, Painless Tennis:
Free Yourself from Pain, Injuries and Limitations,
& Unlock Your Athletic Potential

by David Starbuck Smith

ISBN 978-1-63393-970-7

Published by

◤ köehlerbooks™

210 60th Street
Virginia Beach, VA 23451
800-435-4811
www.koehlerbooks.com

AGELESS
PAINLESS
TENNIS

Free Yourself from Pain,

Injuries and Limitations,

& Unlock Your Athletic Potential

DAVID STARBUCK SMITH

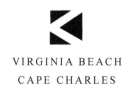

VIRGINIA BEACH
CAPE CHARLES

TABLE OF CONTENTS

EXERCISE REFERENCE

One of my goals is to make it easy for you to follow the exercises and perform them on your own. Therefore, if you want to skip directly to any specific routine I've listed them here for quick and easy reference.

This is typically the place in the book where you'll find a disclaimer of some sort. It would consist of something along the lines of, "Consult your doctor before attempting the exercises..." If you need to consult a physician before doing any of the exercises then please do. If you're not sure then consult one just in case. Keep in mind, although some exercises are recommended for various aches and pains, they're not actually treating the pain—they're treating the underlying postures and misalignments that often result in pain. Nobody knows your body better than you do and you're the boss, so if an exercise doesn't feel right then back off or skip it altogether. Otherwise, enjoy the exercises and the shift they'll produce in your game, your body and your life!

PART I

LAYING THE FOUNDATION

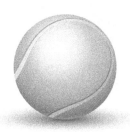

A MESSAGE OF HOPE

I hope this book appeals to every tennis player and athlete of every level and ability around the globe because we all share something in common. Despite our ingenious human design, everyone—regardless of sport, gender, age, ethnicity or athletic skill—develops muscular and postural imbalances.

Tennis players, golfers and baseball players are especially vulnerable to some of these common—and fixable—postural and mechanical imbalances, considering they're all one-sided sports. Runners, cyclists and swimmers also have similar issues even though it falsely appears as if those sports use both sides of the body equally (looks can be deceiving).

Regardless of your preferred sport, I'm betting you have at least six other things in common with every other athlete on the planet:

1. You're tired of nagging injuries that either keep you from playing your best, keep you away from your sport, or keep you from exercising entirely.
2. You'd love to learn a proven and effective method that will help you prevent injury altogether.
3. If you are in pain or injured, rather than wasting precious time, money, and emotional bandwidth on

ten different modalities of treatment, you'd like to find the one technique or cure that works every time.

4. You want to improve your game whether you're a French Open champion or a weekend warrior.

5. You want to continue to play and enjoy your sport for as long as the athletic gods allow.

6. Your muscular and postural imbalances are causing your injuries, keeping you injured, stunting your improvement, impeding your joy of playing, and robbing you of your potential.

What are the signs of these muscular and postural imbalances? Pain anywhere in your body is one obvious indicator, but pain is usually the last manifestation. Before pain sets in, the signs of imbalance are numerous and easily identified. They include shoulders that aren't level, feet that don't point straight ahead, one foot pointing in a different direction from the other, a rounded upper back, a forward head, shorts that look like they sit higher on one hip, shoes that wear unevenly, shifting your weight on one leg all the time while standing, or crossing the same leg over the other when you sit.

On the tennis court they're just as easy to spot: dropping your head on your serve, favoring your forehand over your backhand, moving slower to a wide serve versus one up the middle, not taking your racket back far enough, bending at the waist for a low ball instead of from the hips and knees, struggling to turn your shoulders, falling off balance, hitting the ball too close to you, letting the ball drop too low on your groundstrokes, never coming to net . . . etc.

Although I chose to focus on tennis players, the laws and principles of musculoskeletal imbalance apply to athletes of all sports, and all humans for that matter. If you're a golfer you know you're imbalanced if you lose power on your drive, slice or draw too much, can't line up a putt to save your life or have the touch of a demolition crew wielding a wrecking ball.

Runners, you need this book if you can't boost your mileage without getting injured or overly fatigued, notice one shoe looks like the dog chewed on it while the other still looks relatively new, are a regular track runner or have any kind of nagging pain.

The list goes on and on for every sport.

Other symptoms of a misaligned and imbalanced body include numerous medical ailments. I'm referring to some of the more serious physical consequences of musculoskeletal imbalance that can stop you in your tracks:

- Bulging or ruptured discs in the neck or low back
- Meniscus tears
- Rotator cuff tears
- Osteoarthritis
- Plantar fasciitis
- Achilles tendonitis
- Muscle and joint strains, sprains, and pains

If you're living with chronic injuries and pain, or with any of these painful conditions, this book will not only help you on the tennis court, it might also change your life.

You'll find here one all-encompassing routine to address the five common imbalances shared by almost all humans in one form or another, especially those involved in one-sided sports such as tennis. You'll also discover routines to restore balance and posture, routines to improve flexibility and movement, routines to eliminate pain, routines for overall strength, and routines to boost your performance. All of them will be beneficial. No matter which routine or routines you choose to focus on, my goal is to create an easy and practical approach to getting the most out of your body and your sport.

All the exercises in this book are designed to be done with minimal-to-no equipment, and in the comfort of your home, a gym, on the field or court, or even a hotel room. You'll notice many of the exercises and the accompanying photos illustrating them are repeated throughout the book. This is intentional to limit the number of exercises used in order to make them easier to learn.

Some exercises can also address many different postural conditions and mechanical imbalances at once, regardless of the underlying symptom or condition under which it's listed. For example, I use the downward dog with the knees bent for a lumbar and thoracic spine that doesn't want to move, and with knees straight to link the entire chain of muscles on the back side of your body. In the functional strength chapter, I use it to strengthen the stabilizers of hips and the shoulders. It's the same exercise but it's used for different functions and different purposes.

A few of the exercises will be familiar to you through other therapies you've done including yoga, physical therapy or some other modality of treatment. Reader beware; in this book each exercise is done in a very specific order with a very particular focus on its form that you wouldn't necessarily associate with that exercise. The order and form are therefore important. For this reason, they can easily be downloaded to your computer or your phone so you can have the pictures, instructions and even videos of someone taking you through them.

I'll also show you how to get in touch with your body. With more than fifty-two million Americans taking some form of an anti-inflammatory medication weekly—and that includes just about every tennis player over the age of thirty I've ever met—we're acting as if our aches and pains, our lack of function, and our physical limitations are just normal signs of aging.

They're not. Not even remotely.

Instead, most of our pains and limitations are signs of a body that's out of balance and has begun to deviate from its natural design. That design includes symmetrical shoulders, hips, knees and ankles; I'm going to show you how to reclaim them.

Along with restoring your body back to balance, you're going to lose our culture-perpetuated belief that with age one should feel worse. In fact, whether you're sixty-five or twenty-five, you should feel better than you have in a long, long time.

The first step will be to examine your posture. Faulty posture is like a red-indicator like a warning light in your car. The light flashes red and you know something is either at risk of breaking or is already broken. I'll show you how to read your body's indicator lights and warning signs; then I'll teach you how to be your own mechanic.

Along the way I'll also teach you how to prevent injury, heal pain, increase your longevity, continue to improve your game, and reach your loftiest athletic goals, even if they're as simple as enjoying yourself more and playing into old age.

How? By using unique and revolutionary principles of the *Egoscue Method*®. Time-tested and honed over the last forty years, this highly effective balancing and realignment technique will show you how to tap into your true talent and potential—a potential previously stymied by pain, injury, muscle imbalance, poor joint alignment, lack of flexibility, loss of mobility, or perhaps all of the above.

The *Egoscue Method*® has helped thousands of people cure chronic pain. It's also helped countless numbers of recreational, college and professional athletes of all sports avoid injury and improve their performance.

I was one of them.

Believe me, I know about injury and pain—my own, and yours—based on forty years of playing tennis and twenty years of clinical experience. In that time, I've worked with people of all ages and backgrounds who have exhibited just about every musculoskeletal pain and disability you can imagine.

When I thought about how best to pass on my experience to help as many athletes and tennis players as possible, I looked at the great volume of books already out there and quickly concluded that most of them didn't seem overly practical for the average person just looking to boost their body and their game.

I hope this book is different. I want it to be useable for any tennis player and athlete of any age and skill level. I completely expect the sixty-year-old 3.5 level USTA player, or the golfer with a twenty handicap, to get as much out of it as top-ranked players.

Those of you aspiring to be the best, I want you to be able to tap into the wellspring of talent you were blessed with.

No matter how modest or mighty your aspirations, I want you to feel your best, be able to prevent injury to the best of your ability, fix your current injuries, move better, get stronger, improve your flexibility, and be smarter off the court so you can play your best tennis on it.

I hope you'll allow me to be your guide on this journey, because you're ready to be the ageless and painless athlete you were designed (and destined) to be.

CHAPTER 1

MY PAINFUL BEGINNINGS

I was flat on my back and gasping for air. It was my freshman year on the UC Berkeley tennis team, and I was laid out with the kind of crippling agony that came from the familiar and sudden onset of a massive lower back spasm.

I'd barely covered fifty yards on the track before I collapsed like I'd been stung in the back by an eagle-sized hornet.

The crushing muscle contraction was so intense I couldn't breathe. Finally, after about a minute it released enough for me to get up and run again (think *dumb jock*, not Rhodes Scholar). This time, I managed twenty yards before a subsequent wave of muscle seizures took over and swept me off my feet.

During my freshman year of college, this was just a normal day of running for me (if you can call that running), although the pain didn't just occur when I ran. My back was sore just about every time I played a match or endured a long practice. Sometimes, it hurt just sitting at a desk during class.

College wasn't the first time my body rebelled. I was a high school senior when I encountered my first bout with an injury that wouldn't abate. The tightness started in my hips after a particularly long basketball practice, followed by a few hours of tennis. Being eighteen, I didn't think it was that big of a deal to play varsity basketball for several hours, change clothes, and then play several more hours of intense tennis five days a week. And it wasn't—for about six weeks or so.

One morning I woke up and my legs were so stiff they felt like old and decrepit wooden pegs superglued to cemented hips. Every trepid step threatened to evoke a wave of pain-induced nausea as my hip muscles protested even the slightest movement.

Like most injured young athletes, I figured I would feel better the next day, so I stretched the only way I knew how and tried to wait it out. Three weeks later, it was still nearly impossible for me to move from side to side, and it was unthinkable to sprint without tearing every muscle in my lower body.

Looking back, I should have taken four weeks off all sports, but I was intent on finishing the basketball season while trying to keep up my tennis game. So, like many of you taught to ignore your pain and push on, I gutted through it. *Bad idea.* Never allowing the injury to completely heal, I began to lose to players I had previously beaten with ease. After I lost to the fourth-ranked player on our team in a practice match, my confidence felt as vulnerable and fragile as my body.

This was the first time I had ever felt like an injury was holding me back from my potential. It wouldn't be the last.

My hips eventually recovered, but by the time I started as a freshman at Berkeley, the stiffness had moved to my back. I didn't correlate the two at the time, and despite spending the next three years working with a spate of doctors and trainers, I played almost every match in some degree of discomfort or limitation, while attaining very mixed results.

What I remember most about my college tennis career is frustration. Of course, I loved the team and the travel and the overall experience, but I was almost always playing in pain—physically because of my throbbing back, and emotionally because I agonized over the sense my body was keeping me from playing anywhere near my best tennis.

I was sick of losing to players I believed I could beat, and tired of feeling like my game wasn't improving. I felt helpless as I watched my goals and dreams of becoming one of the best players in the world sabotaged by a body functioning like an out-of-shape ninety-year-old, rather than a happy and healthy twenty-year-old. I felt like the little train that *wanted to*, but just couldn't.

My subsequent experience on the lower levels of the pro tour, mostly competing in satellite events now known as Futures, mirrored my experience in college. I enjoyed my share of fun and some measure of satisfaction at times, but I achieved mixed and often disappointing results while nursing loads of aggravating back pain and a deep sense of powerlessness.

In the end, all I really wanted was an explanation as to why every time I tried to run a lap around a track my lower back would lock up and spasm. I wanted to know why those same muscles stiffened up by every third set. I wanted to know why I grimaced every time I had to bend for a low volley, and why standing around only made my back tighter.

The only answers I heard were the same many of you still hear today—that my low back issues were an indication of tight hamstrings, and weak abs and back muscles. But I knew I could easily palm the ground while bending over to touch my toes, and that I could reel off at least 1,000 sit-ups a day without getting tired, so I *knew* my abs and hamstrings weren't the real issue.

Over time, I decided that these doctors and trainers were giving me a cookie-cutter approach to solving back pain: "Stretch your hamstrings and strengthen your core." But no one *knew* why my back hurt. I finally realized that if I wanted answers, I would have to find them myself. Then I found Pete Egoscue.

CHAPTER 2

LIEUTENANT PETE EGOSCUE

My life unexpectedly changed when my sponsor on the tour told me to go see a fellow named Pete Egoscue, a master and pioneer in the world of anatomical function, posture and pain.

Even today at seventy-four, Pete's a solidly framed six-foot-three-inch-tall retired Marine whose blunt honesty and external gruffness is surpassed only by his compassion for those who require his significant expertise. He had created the *Egoscue Method*® in the early 1970s a few years after suffering a bullet wound to his left hamstring while on tour in Vietnam. After the wound healed, he still endured intense pain in his leg, which the doctors couldn't explain. So they labeled it *post-traumatic stress* and sent him off to a psychiatrist.

Being an extremely stubborn man and a dedicated Marine, Pete disagreed that his inability to walk without pain was in his head, and in the absence of helpful medical guidance he decided he had two choices—either find a way to fix himself or end his life.

Thankfully for the many thousands of people worldwide he has helped both directly and indirectly over the last forty-plus years—including me—he chose the former.

He began by opening an anatomy book. Without any previous anatomy training, the first thing that stood out to him was a picture of the human figure. It seems obvious now, but in the picture the right side of the body looked exactly like the left side.

He knew his didn't.

In fact, his formerly injured and currently painful left leg was severely rotated out while his right leg pointed straight ahead. He postulated that if he could somehow retrain his left leg to point straight ahead again and look like its functional counterpart, maybe he wouldn't have so much pain.

He tirelessly and tenaciously dedicated the next few years to studying the roles of muscles and joints, along with various exercises, and finally devised a routine that began to straighten out his leg.

The straighter it became, the less pain he had, and before long he was back running, jumping and training with the rest of his fellow Marines.

His miraculous turnaround inspired not only his superiors, who promoted him, but also the other soldiers. These men began to approach him asking if he could help them with their various pains. He told them he didn't know anything about pain. However, when he compared them to the anatomy book (the only thing he knew how to do), he noticed their joints didn't line up.

He saw hips that were rotated or swayed forward of the ankles and shoulders, shoulders that were rounded forward, and knees that pointed in while their feet pointed out. He told them he had no idea why they had back pain, or neck pain, or foot pain, or knee pain, but he said that if they restored the position of their bodies to their balanced and symmetrical design just like the anatomical model in his book (the left side of the body should look like the right), maybe, like him, they wouldn't hurt so much.

Thus, began the *Egoscue Method*.

The premise behind Egoscue's method is to treat the position of the body rather than treating the condition of the body. In other words, you have to treat the posture and the position of the joints relative to one another, not just the painful condition. The second premise is to treat the body as a unit rather than solely treating the pieces and parts.

Founded in 1978, *Egoscue Method*® is unique, highly effective, and growing every year, currently with twenty-seven franchised clinics spread over the US, Japan, and Mexico.

Pete plowed his way through a jungle of misinformation, dissent from the medical community, and complex anatomical principles to pave the way for a better understanding of how the human body is connected from head to toe.

Adding my own knowledge and experience to the mix—through a lifelong background in tennis and decades of working with people in pain—I'll lead you down the path he brilliantly set before us toward physical self-discovery and untapped athletic potential.

CHAPTER 3

IT'S YOUR DREAM TO RECLAIM

I remember sitting down with Pete in 1996 and declaring that I was close to throwing in the towel because I wasn't having fun anymore. The pain and constant struggle were slowly but surely stripping me of my joy of tennis.

He looked at me, shook his head and said, "Well, that would be a shame to give up now." I asked why. He replied, "Because you've only been playing with 20 percent of your talent. As it is right now, that's about all your body can access. Once you take that major rotation out of your hips, learn to properly bear weight on your right hip and remove that rounding out of your mid back, you'll actually have a chance to discover how good you can be."

I let those words sink in. I wasn't sure I completely believed Pete then, but for the first time in a very long while I had hope that I might still have a chance of reaching my goals, hope that I could reclaim the dreams of my youth, and hope that I wasn't going to have to give up sports altogether by the time I was twenty-eight because of chronic pain.

What resonated most with me was Pete's explanation for my

pain. He didn't need an X-ray or an MRI. Instead, he took photos of my posture with a standard camera, and my pictures provided all the evidence he needed. Four photos showing the front, both sides, and my back blatantly displayed my flawed posture and the irrefutable imbalance. With Pete's help, I could see the right hip rotation, the excessive forward rounding in my mid back, the torque in my lower right leg, and my right shoulder blade sitting higher than my left.

Although shocking, seeing my postural imbalances for the first time was also somehow inspiring. Staring at the crooked guy in the pictures, and knowing it was possible to change, reignited my desire to chase my dreams. With nothing to lose, I dove into the exercises with hopeful enthusiasm.

The exercises Pete and his crew took me through were surprisingly simple. Some were passive and used gravity to do all the work while others were extremely active and engaged all my joints and muscles at once. Many of the exercises were unique and products of Pete's anatomical mind; others were familiar. The exercises I had encountered before, either in physical therapy or yoga, were used in a different way than I was accustomed. The goal wasn't to stretch or strengthen my back muscles, or even to treat my back, but instead to realign my entire body from head to toe using exercises specifically targeted to my postural and mechanical imbalances.

I admit I was both worried and somewhat skeptical it was going to work. After all the time, money, effort, multiple doctors and numerous physical therapists I had seen, the possibility crossed my mind that nothing would change. After all, what could Pete possibly know that all of them didn't?

It turns out he knew a lot. Three weeks after diligently doing my exercises, I put my running shoes on and set off to test Pete's method along with my back. I ran five miles with no pain for the first time in eight years. Running felt so good I didn't want to stop.

That run was a revelation. It was definitive proof something had changed, and I wasn't irreparably *broken* after all.

The next revelation came on the tennis court. I reacted faster, I moved more fluidly to the ball, I felt more on balance and stable when I got to it, and I wasn't spraining my ankles anymore.

I felt freedom. Freedom from pain, freedom from feeling like I was playing every match with a disadvantage. Freedom from the constant physical and emotional struggle. It was as if the sealed vault of athletic possibility opened again and infused me with renewed enthusiasm to pursue my dreams.

Off the court, liberated from the pain, I was able to train harder than ever with no ill effects. Incorporating longer runs, cone drills and hill sprints without inciting back spasms added a new dimension to my training routine and it all paid off. Within a few months, I played the four best tournaments of my adult life and reached the finals of an invitational doubles tournament that gave me a split of $70,000 in prize money.

I was finally living up to the potential I always believed I possessed.

Then something unexpected happened. Six months after finishing Pete's program, reaching the finals of the doubles tournament, and playing the best tennis of my life, I felt like there was nothing more to prove to myself, or to anyone else. I had finally accomplished what I set out to do—to feel whole again, to become a professional tennis player, and to enjoy the game I love. I had found peace, and with it the readiness to move on to the next chapter of my life.

Weeks later, I played my final tournament in St. Louis, Missouri.

I had always known there would be life after tennis, but I'll never forget my last match. I had just won the first set against a formidable player in the third round when I sat on the changeover and realized, for the first time in my life, that I didn't care if I won or lost. It was an unexpected epiphany, yet somewhat welcome clarity that it was time to walk away. So, I lost the next two sets, packed my bags, and flew home.

Without tennis as my driving motivation anymore, I formed new goals. They were simple: Learn as much as I could about human anatomy, help others living with pain, and aid those frustrated souls whose athletic potential was being hijacked by their own imbalanced bodies.

I made the decision to return to Berkeley to finish my degree in integrative biology/pre-med and then went back to Pete's clinic in San Diego to try to learn as much as I could about pain and the human body. I wanted to know what he knew. I wanted to learn everything I could about anatomical function, about pain, and about how to solve it.

That's my story. I included it because I'm sure you can relate through similar experiences or frustrations, and I wanted to give you some context for the upcoming chapters and exercises. From here on out—with the exception of a few personal anecdotes to add some color and to illustrate some key concepts—it's all about you. It's time to free your mind and body so you can play without limitations.

PART II
A NEW WAY OF THINKING

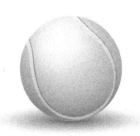

CHAPTER 4

THE AGE-OLD EXCUSE

All tennis players and athletes age, and everyone nurses the occasional injury. But are those injuries due to age? I've worked with thousands of people over the years, and I'm still astounded by the common rationale many of us are conditioned to use to explain away our aches and pains or poor performance.

Three major scapegoats attract the lion's share of the blame, not just in my clinic or on the tennis court, but in our modern American culture:

1. Age
2. Genetics
3. The sport itself

Age

We're conditioned to believe that pain, injury, and progressive weakness are normal milestones of aging. In fact, age is the most common fall guy for many doctors, health professionals, and humans in general to explain the *why* of our physical status or poor performance. Yet, blaming your age is just a story you tell yourself that's seldom true.

After all, how do you know your injury or your decreased performance is age-related?

The presumption itself is detrimental to your game and your health because it enables you to avoid digging any deeper for an answer as to why the pain or weakness is present.

Furthermore, the belief that age leads to injury and weakness unfairly victimizes all of us by evolving into an all-encompassing case of *that's just the way it is*, the ultimate blow-off that transfers the responsibility of our health to fate.

The same goes for genetics. Obviously, we can't help getting older, or our genetic makeup. So, if pain or injury is a product of either, then what can we do?

I like to address the age fallacy straight-away with every person I work with. Obviously, if you get hit by a bus or tackled by a 350-pound human with a helmet, the reason for the pain is clear—your knee was demolished by an immovable object. Traumatic injury aside, the first question I'll pose to you is, *Why do you think you hurt?* The question itself sheds light on your underlying belief system about the root cause of your pain.

Now go even deeper and ask yourself, *What do I believe, really believe, is the cause of my pain or physical limitation?* What's the deep-down fear you hold about the cause? That it's just age and beyond your control? That there is something undiagnosed and irretrievably broken? There are no right or wrong answers, but there are limiting stories and detrimental beliefs that guide your actions, and thus your outcomes.

In other words, if you believe the pain is out of your hands, then at least subconsciously you might be less inclined to put your heart and soul into any kind of therapy or treatment since you ultimately feel you can't be helped.

That doesn't necessarily mean you won't be helped, but if the first treatment you try doesn't work, then you might be easily discouraged and chalk it up to an unfixable problem.

On the other hand, if you knew you were fixable, that belief might lead to a very different set of actions and results.

Either way, some beliefs are more empowering than others.

Of course, the underlying belief I often hear is, "I think I'm just getting old."

If that was your response, you're in good company. However, like any story we tell ourselves, it's always helpful to break it down and examine its validity.

Think about it. If your right knee hurts, and age is the underlying culprit, then how old is your left knee or ankle, hip, or shoulder?

I can hear you chuckling. It's humorous because, suddenly, passing the pain off on age doesn't make much sense.

The same is true for pain on both sides of your neck or back. I recently worked with a client named Mary who came in looking for relief from her back pain. She thought her back pain was a sign and symptom of getting old; she was fifty-six years young at the time. When responding to my question of when she felt pain, she would reply, "It comes and goes." I countered with the question, "Mary, if your back pain is related to age and it comes and goes, do you suddenly become twenty again when it's gone?"

She laughed and acknowledged that her age didn't suddenly drop thirty-six years. My point was not to make fun of her. It was simply to get her to examine her beliefs, and to ask herself if the story she's been using to rationalize her symptom for all these years made sense.

Another problem with the belief that age is at fault is that we can't do anything about it. We're all aging, and with some luck and conscious self-care, we're going to continue to age. If we blame everything we feel on getting older, we're just relinquishing our power, and with it our responsibility for our bodies and our health. No matter what your age, my suggestion is to dismiss this belief because it isn't serving you well. It never has, and never will.

The truth is, you might feel old because you're in pain, but you're not in pain because you're old.

Of course, television has a way of reminding us how we're supposed to feel as we get older. How many commercials peddling back braces, or nonsteroidal anti-inflammatory drugs like aspirin, or the latest miracle drug (with fifty side effects that are worse than the condition it treats) do we see on TV that subliminally declare we should feel progressively weaker, more tired, and increasingly sore with each passing year?

Commercials are just one of many sources of misleading information. I generally like listening to most tennis commentators, but I was disappointed listening to one of them during Roger Federer's Grand Slam matches in 2016 because after just about every unforced error he would say something like, "Those thirty-five-year-old legs just don't quite get to the ball like they used to."

It seemed that every time Fed made an error it had something to do with him getting older, insinuating that his age was making him slower, or weaker, or less accurate. Then, the next year, at the crippling old age of thirty-six, Fed went 52-5 with seven titles that included the Australian Open and Wimbledon. If that's what old age brings, I want more of it.

Of course, that particular commentator isn't the only one guilty of perpetuating the age-is-athletic-doom stereotype. If you listen long enough to just about any sportscaster from any sport, at some point they'll associate a player's age with diminished performance, or speak in awe at how well the athlete is playing considering they're thirty-seven. The message is clear; any normal thirty-seven-year-old should be content with what he's accomplished and should probably be sitting on the sidelines watching someone younger win.

Luckily for us tennis fans, in a sport where turning thirty supposedly meant it was time to pack up the rackets and bust out the crossword puzzles, legendary players like Federer, Rafael Nadal, Venus and Serena Williams, and hosts of others are making the case that thirty-plus is nowhere near the beginning of the end. In fact, all these world-class athletes are showing their age by kicking younger and much less experienced butt. They're changing the age paradigm of the sport by making the case that older might just be better.

One more thing about age before I let the topic, uh, rest. Your body doesn't keep track of your birthdays. When we hit that magic year of sixty, our body doesn't suddenly decide, "Well, I'm sixty, time to pile on some leg pain, maybe a little arthritis, and a side of gout."

More often than not, we do that to ourselves based on our preconceived and repeatedly conditioned beliefs about what comes with age. Pain and other health challenges can be a self-fulfilling prophecy if you believe, as I do, in the great power of the mind.

Genetics

A few years ago, I was able to work with a brilliant young woman who'd just finished her PhD in chemistry at Harvard. The first time we met she was on crutches due to ankle and foot pain and had already sought the advice of every foot and ankle doctor she could find. They believed, based on the X-rays and their evaluations, that her ankle pain was coming from bone spurs and weak ankles.

As a result of their counsel, at twenty-five years old she had already endured two surgeries to try to fix what they thought to be the problem. She was also led to believe that running was out of the question, and she was resigned to never run again.

When I asked her why she thought she had the pain, she said, "Well, my father had tennis elbow, so . . ."

I let that hang for a few seconds because I was trying to grasp the connection. With further prodding, she explained that she thought her ankle pain was the result of loose and weak ligaments and tendons. She continued to reason that her father must have also had weak ligaments and tendons because, after all, he had tennis elbow. After taking all that in, I grew a big smile because I finally understood.

Her underlying reasoning to justify the pain was genetics. So, I asked her, "Does the pain come and go?"

"Yes."

"How do genetics account for that?"

She paused. "I'm not sure."

"Okay, if the pain is on one side and it's due to genetics, is your good ankle from your mother's side?

She laughed. "You're a jerk."

"I know, but you're a scientist and I'm just trying to use logic and reason here to examine your hypothesis. Last question: Do you really think there's a gene that codes for tennis elbow?"

She laughed again. "Probably not."

"Agreed. I'm no genetic scientist, but I'm guessing there isn't one."

"Okay, okay, so what do you think is wrong with my ankle?"

I explained that I believed the condition of her ankle— deteriorating cartilage, strained ankle ligaments, bone spurs and pain—was due to the *position* of her ankle. Her collapsed ankle position had to do with her internally rotated knee and imbalanced hip muscles. I proved it when I had her stand and pay attention to where her weight was on that foot.

It was all on the inside where the pain was. I then had her put her hands behind her head with her elbows back and told her to walk, which was a way of temporarily realigning her hips and spine. Her ankle came back toward neutral and she suddenly had no pain. So much for genetics as the culprit.

It didn't take long before she was rock climbing, hiking, and walking with no pain, and she now runs without a second thought. The key to her recovery had very little to do with the exercises I gave her. It was her change in belief that she could heal that made all the difference.

Let's imagine for a second that pain and limitation are, in fact, genetic. I'm sure it's possible and happens in some cases, but ask yourself these questions: Do you think your body can still change? For example, do you think that by lifting weights you can get stronger, or by running enough you can look like a runner? Of course, the answers are yes.

Your body abides by the laws of adaptation. With the right stimulus, you can go from having the body of a moldy couch potato to having the physique of Arnold Schwarzenegger at his prime. It all depends on the stimulus you choose to give yourself.

The point is, you can change despite your genetics, and you will, no matter how much your mother's back hurts, or the severity of your father's tennis elbow.

Again, I want to point out that when you use genetics or age as an explanation for the *why* of pain, you take away your responsibility and your power to identify the root cause. I know you wouldn't be reading this book if you really believed you were powerless to change, but I make the point just in case there's still a lingering belief, or a small fear lurking inside you, that pain is an inevitable part of life, and you're just going to have to live with it.

No, you don't.

The Sport or Activity

The third most common refrain I hear to explain aches and pains is to blame the sport or activity itself. "Tennis hurt my back," or "Running is bad for me." The underlying belief is that your body hurts because the activity made it hurt. If that's true, were you running or playing tennis on just the ankle or knee that ended up hurting? I'm guessing you were running and playing tennis on both legs.

Humans are designed to run. We're designed to jump, twist, turn, swing a golf club, crush forehands, and lunge for volleys. The activity or movement you made when you got hurt or injured wasn't the problem. For one thing, you've probably done that activity a hundred or a thousand times in the past without issue. So why now?

The problem isn't the activity, *it's the body you're bringing to the activity.*

Chances are, you're bringing an imbalanced and somewhat dysfunctional body to everything you do. The sport—tennis, golf, running, whatever—is asking for more function than your shoulder or back or knee is able to provide at the moment because they're out of balance and out of position. We break at our weakest points, and pain is the resulting consequence.

When you do the self-assessment in this book, you'll start to discover what those weak and overstressed points are so you can tackle them head-on.

CHAPTER 5

THE MYTH OF OSTEOARTHRITIS

There's another common age-related myth I want to address—osteoarthritis. The most common belief is that arthritis is due to old age. It's not. Again, how old is your other knee that is less arthritic or not arthritic at all?

Let's start with what arthritis actually is. In Latin, *arthra* translates into *joint*, and *itis* translates into *inflammation*. So, arthritis literally means *inflammation of the joint*. Inflammation is the body's healthy and natural response to tissue irritation or damage. Arthritis occurs when the bones that comprise the joint don't align correctly.

For example, a knee becomes arthritic when the upper and lower leg bones are misaligned to the point that it causes the cartilage (the knee's shock-absorbing bumper guard) to wear away unevenly. Eventually, the cartilage in the affected area deteriorates enough that it loses its ability to protect against the friction generated from the motion in the joint. The result is tissue irritation and inflammation, commonly diagnosed by doctors as arthritis.

In addition, since the misalignment impedes the function of the knee, the surrounding muscles, tendons and ligaments can also be irritated or damaged, which further increases the inflammation.

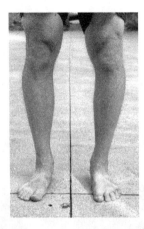 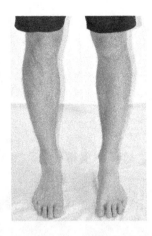

Figure 5.1. Observe the bowing of the lower legs which result in the ankles collapsing to counterbalance. The bowing creates a misalignment in the knee joint putting all the stress on the inside of the knee.

Figure 5.2. A much more neutral alignment of the upper and lower legs, and thus more evenly distributed stress through the knee.

However, the medical world commonly calls osteoarthritis a degenerative joint *disease* rather than a common and fixable response to misalignment, so many people just live with it like it's a fact of life.

Allow me to show you how misalignment can create tissue damage. First, make your hands into fists and press your knuckles together like your hands are punching each other (*Fig. 5.1*). Align your knuckles in the grooves in the opposite hand. Next, push your fists together and feel how the pressure is generally evenly distributed on each fist as you push.

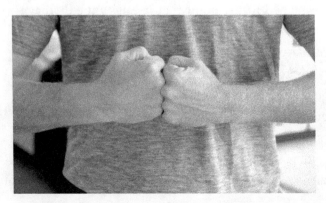

Figure 5.3 Knuckles aligned in grooves

Now take your knuckles out of the grooves, align them directly on the other knuckles (*Fig. 5.2*), and press again. Notice how uncomfortable the pressure becomes because now you're pressing all the weight of your fist into just one or two knuckles.

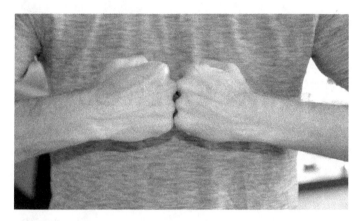

Figure 5.4 Knuckles misaligned

Now rub them back and forth. Ouch. Imagine doing that all day; it won't take long to develop skin irritation followed by pain and eventually damage to your fingers.

Your knee, or hip, or shoulder became arthritic in the same way. Misaligned bones exert too much pressure on one part of the joint rather than distributing equal pressure throughout. Your body is coming to the rescue to heal the damage by creating inflammation of your joint, a.k.a. *arthritis.*

The solution is to trigger your muscles to realign the bones and joints. Once the bones are aligned, the pressure on the joint will be more evenly distributed, your cartilage will stop deteriorating, and the arthritis you suspected was a result of age will magically disappear even though you're getting older by the day.

CHAPTER 6

THE THREE *M'S* FOR ENERGY

The quality of your life, and your tennis game, is often dictated by your energy level. Not only is it tough to imagine gutting out a three-setter, but it's difficult to feel focused, loving, excited, joyful, and grateful when you're tired. It's also difficult to pursue an exciting career, cultivate a relationship, or create a new business opportunity when you're exhausted by the daily grind of life.

So how do you find more energy on and off the court? One way is to have a balanced, and thus energy-efficient, musculoskeletal system which you'll restore by doing the exercises in this book. The other helpful alternatives are the three *M*'s—meditation, metabolism, and motion.

Meditation

In terms of meditation, I advocate three minutes a day to recharge and replenish your energy and your spirit. Yes, that's all. Three minutes a day will change your life and help you on the tennis court. That is, as long as you disconnect from your fears and anxieties that are stripping you of your energy and life-force. You need three minutes to just *be*. Here's how:

Meditation 1

Find a comfortable seated position and breathe. Inhale and let your stomach extend and fill with air; exhale and feel your stomach empty. The goal is to engage your diaphragm, so try not to breathe from your chest. Clear your mind and focus on breathing this way for three minutes, allowing your diaphragm and lungs to expand and contract. That's it.

Meditation 2

This time you focus on a feeling like gratitude or love. Start the timer and think about something you're grateful for and let the feelings of gratitude fill you. Feel it, breathe it, and let it expand inside you for three minutes. You can be grateful for your parents, your partner, the beauty of a shimmering lake, or your beating heart that continues to give you life. Focusing on the positive feeling derived from something or someone meaningful to you will disconnect you from any fear and negativity that can surround your space and drain you of energy.

There are two reasons these meditations work. First, it's impossible to feel fear, anger, worry or anxiety when you're feeling gratitude (or love) or when you're in the moment and focused completely on your breath. Second, time is an illusion.

Three minutes will feel like three hours to many of you when you actually submerse yourself in the experience. You will come away feeling more rested, you'll have increased mental clarity, and you'll definitely have more energy to employ on and off the court.

Metabolism

Your metabolic rate is essentially a measurement of the number of calories you burn while hanging out on your couch. It's also an indicator of the amount of energy your body is producing. Generally speaking, the higher your metabolic rate, the healthier you are, the more energy you have, and the better you feel. On the other hand, the slowing of your metabolic rate can lead to major physical repercussions. Weight gain, muscle loss and weakness, heart disease, and the onset of diabetes are just some of the common and ugly consequences.

There are two fireproof ways to gain energy and impact your metabolic rate—eat cleaner food and move more. I was not-so-subtly reminded of both when I stopped playing tennis.

Three months into my first full-time job, I gained eighteen pounds and didn't even know it until I stepped on the scale for the first time. Surprise would be putting it mildly since it was the first time in my life I realized I could actually gain weight. I should have known it was possible since I was no longer playing tennis all day, but it never even occurred to me that becoming the poster child for the Pillsbury Dough Boy was within my reach.

Of course, devouring half a box of Wheat Thins smeared with cream cheese almost every day after work didn't help.

Although not recommended for everyone, my crazy solution to my newly acquired waist size was to sign up for my first half-Ironman triathlon.

I'd never been a long-distance runner, definitely never been into biking, and had swum my first lap ever only a few years earlier, yet I thoroughly enjoyed the challenge. Unlike a tennis tournament, my goal was to finish rather than to win. It felt somewhat liberating to just enjoy the training and the process without any pressure to perform.

Although you definitely don't have to do triathlons to change your metabolism, if you're embarking on a new physical endeavor, I suggest doing it purely for the fun and challenge rather than the result. I also suggest using the "I wasn't really trying to win" disclaimer any time your significant other finishes ahead of you, as mine did in the race (which I never lived down).

Of course, training for a triathlon, or exercising in general to boost your metabolic rate, requires energy.

Yet, after sitting at work for eight to ten hours a day and eating processed food that sucks the life out of us, it's no wonder many people would rather kick up their feet and tune out to reruns of *Law and Order* than go for a long walk. The unfortunate consequence is that our bellies, our deteriorating health, and pain become reflections of a metabolism that's revving more like an old scooter than the Formula 1 race car it's designed to be.

The good news is that we can change quickly, since burning energy in our bodies is not like burning gas in a car. If you drive a car and use up gas one day, the next time you drive you start with less gas than you had the day before. The body is the opposite.

When you exercise and use energy, after enough rest, the next time you exercise you have more energy than you did before. Expending energy begets more energy because our heart, lung and muscle cells adapt to become more efficient.

In terms of food, efficiency in both a car and your body will be bolstered by using cleaner fuel, so drop the processed stuff and eat real food.

Motion

There's a major anatomical law by which every living organism and every human on the planet abides. *The less activity we do, the weaker we get, and the more activity we do, the stronger we get*, at just about any age. It's that simple.

We've all used the saying that "nobody's perfect." We should have said, "Nobody's perfect after the age of six or seven." In truth, almost all children between the ages of one to six exhibit extraordinarily perfect posture and symmetry, not to mention total and balanced function. Their shoulders, hips, knees and ankles stack up and they have perfect S-curves in their spines.

Kids often begin to lose their perfect symmetry when they must spend long hours sitting at a desk chair at school. Essentially, we all begin to lose it when we stop moving constantly. Kids never stop moving unless they're about to fall asleep or they're taking a break to fuel up for more moving; they bend, twist, turn, do cartwheels, sit on their heels to look at a bug, climb over everything and everyone, crawl everywhere, and a million other movements that take their muscles and joints through a full range of motion and function.

School, although intellectually stimulating, isn't always physically stimulating. Sitting at a desk puts the kibosh on motion for many hours. Those hours add up and our bodies adapt to the non-moving just as it did to the moving. It's called the *law of adaptation,* and it's one of the major reasons we're still here after six million-plus years. It's also the reason why we can get our bodies back to where we started; our bodies will adapt to the new functional stimulus the exercises in this book are designed to provide.

The fancy term for adaptation is *neuroplasticity.* Simply put, our brains and our bodies not only can change, but they change constantly. We are literally in a constant state of evolution. Every second of every day our bodies are responding to the air we breathe, the nutrients we eat (or don't eat), and the motion we receive, whether good stimulus or bad. Unfortunately, as a culture, we seem to be adapting to less and less motion as technology continues to progress.

The recently popular catchphrase among health professionals is, "*Sitting is the new smoking, only it will kill you quicker.*" That statement is only partially true. I don't think the problem is sitting, but rather the lack of moving. I believe if you get enough motion in your life you can sit for long hours without repercussion (after all, you got away with it for years). That's not to say sitting all day is good for you; it isn't. Without enough joint and cardiovascular motion to counterbalance it, sitting all day could work like a slow-moving cancer. It can gradually lead to a deterioration in function and chronic pain as your living and breathing cells are starved from positive and varied stimulus. Imagine being stuck in a box for hours, days and years and how that would affect your body. That's how little motion many of us get on a daily basis.

However, unlike some very unfortunate cancers, the *sitting condition* is almost entirely reversible with the renewal of varied and plentiful motion. The first step is to acknowledge our habits.

Think about a common day for many of us in the twenty-first century. We wake up and sit to eat, we sit in the car on the way to work, we sit at our desks for six to ten hours with minimal breaks, we go to the gym and sit on an exercise bike, we drive home and sit down for dinner, and then we saunter over to the couch for a few hours of sitting in front of the television.

What kind of stimulus is the body getting? *Imbalanced stimulus* because it's almost all in the form of flexion (the muscles on the front side of the body are in a shortened position all day) similar to being stuck in that box.

As the body adapts to all this flexion, the extensor muscles—those on the back side of the body—begin to atrophy, throwing the delicate postural balance out of whack. The spine begins to change its shape, and then we go play tennis or head out for a run.

You've heard the term *weekend warrior.* I think the more applicable term is *weakened warrior* because without a balanced, mobile and fully functioning musculoskeletal system you're charging the battlefield without your most potent weapon. It's like Joan of Arc taking on an army with a wooden spoon while riding a Shetland pony. The difference is the enemy is the normal physical stress and the demand that sport confers on your body rather than blood-thirsty soldiers.

The point is, we need the kind of plentiful and varied motion that sitting on our butts all day can't provide. When we don't have that motion, we pay the penalty of injury, pain, and limitation.

Ever wonder why so many doctors and studies claim that once we turn forty, we can begin to lose up to 5 percent of our muscle mass every year? Because they're observing a general population that moves less and less as the days and months pass by, and that our bodies are withering from the lack of motion and physical demand.

Ask yourself, *Do I move as much now as I did when I was a kid?* Of course not. Most of us have full-time jobs, kids of our own, and busy lives. We're simply moving less than we once did before our adult lives took over.

The truth is, we are move-it-or-lose-it creatures, and some of us aren't movin' it enough. Although incorrectly correlating aging to weakness, scientific studies bolster this notion.

I'm not saying you must move all the time or that you can't have a normal life. I'm not even suggesting you need to run marathons, or repeatedly blast your biceps with weights. I *am* suggesting that if you want to get stronger at any age and gain muscle mass, then start moving more, and increase your current physical stimulus.

The *Totally Balanced Tennis* routine will be a big first step.

In addition, you can join a yoga class, walk forward, backward, and sideways up a hill and then back down instead of your usual walk, or take swing dancing lessons with your partner. Whatever you do, use your imagination and don't settle for health that's merely good enough.

With a little work, you can be the poster adult for the argument that you can still be strong, feel great, and have tremendous life and energy at your age.

Or at any age.

CHAPTER 7

MUSCLE IMBALANCE— THE ENEMY OF YOUR POTENTIAL

C onsidering your goal is to feel your best and to be your best in your sport, I can't state strongly enough that imbalance is the true nemesis of your athletic talent and potential, your longevity in the sport, your enjoyment, and your ability to remain injury-free. By imbalance, I mean musculoskeletal imbalance, the unfortunate union of muscle imbalance and skeletal misalignment. For quick reference, I often use the simple term *imbalance* to encompass musculoskeletal imbalance, and overall postural misalignment.

Muscular imbalance is the result of some muscles being too tight, too short, too weak, too strong, too loose, or too anything in relation to the other muscles around a joint. Skeletal misalignment occurs when your bones and joints are out of position and your posture is skewed. Muscle imbalance always leads to skeletal misalignment because muscles move bones and joints. It's also possible for the reverse to be true when a joint is knocked out of place due to an outside force or trauma. However, in my experience, 99 percent of the time the imbalance originates from the muscles due to our past injuries, habits, sports, and routines.

You simply can't play your very best tennis over a period of days, weeks, or months with a major imbalance. Most of us aren't playing our very best tennis today because of it. Why? In a word, *compensation.*

Imbalance leads to *over-compensation* from other muscles and joints, inefficient movement, wasted energy, and it often results in muscle or joint injury. Muscles literally bleed excess energy when compensating for another muscle, and muscles, tendons, and ligaments aren't designed to do another muscle's job over the long haul. Therefore, it's only a matter of time before those other structures break down and fatigue sooner than they should and become susceptible to pain and/or injury. Obviously, pain and injury would keep anyone from reaching their top potential.

In order to illustrate the effects of imbalance and the resulting compensation, I'll tell you Susan's story. She was age forty and has a postural condition where her upper back and shoulders noticeably rounded forward (*Fig. 7.1*). One effect of this fixable condition (and there are multiple effects) is that it compromised the ability of Susan's shoulder and upper back to reach the correct position while serving.

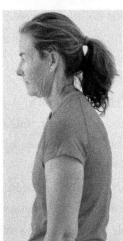

Since her upper back wasn't moving enough to allow her to reach up for the ball, her lower back tried to make up for the lack of motion by over-arching.

Miraculously, she was able to pull it off for years, but eventually her lower back muscles had enough. One day, Susan went out to play a league match with her club team, tossed the ball in the air to serve, reached up to hit it, and her lower back locked up so hard she had to be carried off the court.

Figure 7.1 Noticeable rounding in the upper back

Susan had suffered from lower back pain, but it easily could have been her shoulder that was injured if her lower back decided not to move either. I suspect that would have come next if she hadn't come to me. She likely would've treated the lower back pain only—not the cause.

And to protect her low back the next time she played, she would have used her shoulder to generate all the motion and power for her serve.

As soon as we addressed the position and function of her upper back, her lower back relaxed and she went back to playing without pain.

What Susan hadn't realized even before her back injury was how much excess energy her body had to expend every time she stepped on the court. All her back and shoulder muscles were fatiguing quickly by working overtime to compensate for her lack of function. Her muscles were leaking excess energy like left-on headlights draining a car battery. Susan's scenario was all too common.

If your alignment is compromised by muscle imbalance, and I guarantee it is, you're expending unnecessary energy to get your body in the most functional position to hit any stroke, or to maintain your running, cycling or swimming form.

I'm sure you know from experience that as soon as your muscles fatigue, you're more vulnerable to injury, poor footwork, and the early-onset mental fatigue that always follows physical decline. None of which are a recipe for success.

I mentioned earlier that Susan's shoulder might have been next in line for injury. Many of you are also bringing a rounded shoulder (or shoulders) to the tennis court, and a series of different compensations are taking place in your elbow and wrist.

All sports require a large amount of function from all your joints, especially tennis, which is one of the reasons it's such a great sport to maintain speed, strength and stimulation to your whole body. However, your rounded shoulder can't function optimally and efficiently when it's out of its neutrally aligned position. The reason is the prime movers and force producers of your shoulder aren't able to work together as a unit, and they effectively become weaker.

Those larger shoulder muscles then have to abdicate their job to your smaller and weaker wrist, elbow, and rotator cuff muscles.

The body is incredibly resilient, but serve enough times using the wrong muscles, and trouble is sure to follow. It should come as no surprise that when it comes time to ramp up your serve for a big point, you suddenly pop a rotator cuff muscle, or experience a sharp pain in your elbow, or tweak a ligament in your wrist because those parts couldn't take the strain of the demand any longer.

We often blame tennis for these injuries or bouts of pain, but they were just accidents waiting to happen due to a misaligned shoulder joint.

On the other hand, a balanced and functional shoulder can handle that extra effort in a pressure situation, and you're rewarded with a monster serve that makes you feel like John Isner or Serena Williams, even if only for a brief moment.

There are other repercussions from imbalance besides expending excess energy and potential injury. A lack of functional alignment may also keep you from getting your knees, hips, and spine in the ideal position to create power, maintain balance, or even to produce touch and finesse.

For instance, while a shoulder joint lacking full range of motion and function prohibits you from getting the most out of your serve, it also limits the backswing and follow-through of every groundstroke.

A quick story highlighting imbalance as it relates to power: I've been working with a highly ranked national junior player who verbally committed to one of the top tennis colleges in the country. His father complained that his son just didn't seem to have enough power on his serve, and he was worried that he wasn't going to be able to physically keep up with the older college players.

He was right, but not for the reason he thought. He believed his son had to work out on weights to get stronger and to hit a bigger serve. I took one look at this very talented kid and knew that lifting weights wasn't going to help, because strength had nothing to do with his weak serve. Instead, his rotated right hip was the culprit.

One look at his abducted (turned out) right foot and medial (rotated in) right knee told me he had a problem properly keeping weight on his right hip. Then I saw him serve. As he bent his knees before attempting to explode up to the ball, his right knee collapsed in toward the left. When his knee collapsed inward, his base of support abandoned him, and all he had left to generate any power on the ball was his arm (*Fig. 7.2*). Hopefully, by now you can guess where the kid was also complaining of pain: his elbow and wrist.

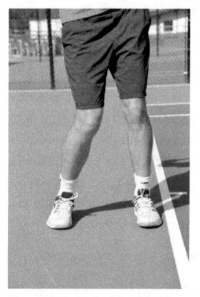

Figure 7.2 Example of the right hip not bearing proper load during a serve

If he had a more functional right hip, his joints would have remained aligned, allowing the muscles in his bent legs to load up all their potential energy. That energy would then be properly and completely transferred to his upper body as his legs exploded up toward the ball, and finally released through his arm and racket. The result would have been a much faster and more powerful serve, and much less stress on his arm.

The fix came down to taking the rotation out of his right hip and strengthening the correct hip muscles (rather than lifting weights) to allow the smooth and efficient transfer of power from a body that was aligned and working together as a unit.

All power and balance in just about any sport originates from the hips, so any hip imbalance or lack of function is going to detract from one's ability to stay balanced on the run, or to generate maximum power on your serve or groundstrokes. Imbalanced hips also don't allow you to move equally to each side, nor can you load your front foot properly when you hit a backhand compared to a forehand.

You've experienced the effects of imbalanced hips if you've ever pulled up early on your backhand or shanked a shot from not staying down long enough.

Shanking is often the result of an improper weight transfer from your back leg to your front leg. The reason for the lack of complete weight transfer is a subconscious (neurological) unwillingness to fully load your front leg. Thus, you pull up early instead of staying down.

The same scenario applies when you find yourself turning out of your forehand early, or if you're having trouble finding the timing on your serve. Often, they're both signs of hips that aren't balanced and of one leg that's bearing more than its share of the weight.

Do you ever find yourself bending your back instead of your knees for low balls (*Fig. 7.3*)? It's a sign that your lower back is compensating for tight or weak hip muscles, and again, you're not transferring weight properly and evenly to your front leg. Do you like moving wide for a slice serve on the deuce court but not so much for a kick serve in the ad court? That's because of an overloaded left hip in your return stance. That same overloaded left hip applies if you're a righty and you prefer moving to your forehand side rather than your backhand.

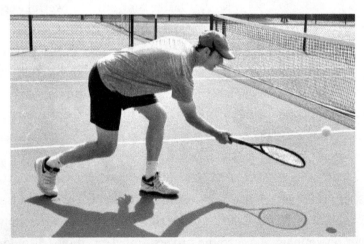

Figure 7.3 Bending for a low volley with your back instead of your knees

The examples of musculoskeletal dysfunction and how it affects your tennis game are endless, and so are the consequences. Pain and injury are consequences for sure, but so is winning and losing.

Considering tennis is a game of milliseconds and inches, wins or losses are often decided by just a few points. Shanking your forehand at a key moment or getting to that wide serve just a little slower because you're loaded unevenly, or fatiguing faster than you should because you're bleeding excess energy, determines winners and losers every day.

The good news is that *all* of it is fixable or preventable. Stated another way, the overwhelming satisfaction of feeling your best and getting the most out of your body is not only doable but inevitable when you first identify, then attack, your own musculoskeletal issues.

CHAPTER 8

SYMPTOM OR CAUSE? A MAJOR MISUNDERSTANDING

One of the major shortcomings of the Western medical model, commonly called *allopathic care*, that we follow here in the United States is that symptoms are often misunderstood. We treat symptoms as if they were the cause.

Take an example of a painful wrist. Most doctors and health professionals would treat the wrist without addressing the rounded and forward shoulder—often the real cause—that almost always accompanies it. Even a rounded shoulder could be a symptom of an opposite hip dysfunction, but that's never treated or even looked at because the symptom was misunderstood and treated alone.

The result is that you've rested your painful wrist, and you've received the best treatment from the best therapists and doctors, and it feels better. However, since you haven't solved the underlying cause, you end up right back where you started, with a malfunctioning shoulder or hip that still needs to be remedied before it causes more symptoms to pop up somewhere else.

My journey led me to many different doctors, trainers, and physical therapists. Their diagnosis was that there was something wrong with my back, my ankle, and my hips, and that they all needed to be examined and treated independently. I did have a disc herniation and a strained ankle ligament, but they were just symptoms of misalignment—not causes.

I know now the disc bulge was just a symptom of a rotated pelvis and of imbalanced spinal muscles that once remedied would allow the disc to go back in place.

It took a lot of years of pain, stress, and frustration, but when I finally found the helpful guidance I was seeking, I came to understand my back pain, my ankle sprain, and other ailments were all connected by the same musculoskeletal imbalance that was obvious by just looking in the mirror. All those ailments were symptoms of a misaligned body.

More importantly, I learned how to fix those misalignments and imbalances myself.

When I finally recognized and treated the cause, the aggravating symptoms disappeared like gnats in the wind, and I began to play the best tennis of my life.

The point I wish to drive home is that the pain didn't signal something wrong with my back. It was a message that there was something wrong with the *position* of my back, just like there was something wrong with the position of my hips and the position of my ankle.

In the *Egoscue* clinics we have a saying: "The problem isn't the condition of your body—the disc herniation, the ankle pain, the neck pain, and other pain conditions—it's the *position* of your body."

Treat the position, and the painful conditions typically take care of themselves because they are almost always just symptoms of misalignment. By restoring muscle balance and the natural, neutral alignment of your body, you can fix the cause of the pain.

We have another saying. "You can repair or replace a worn-out tire, but until you fix the alignment of the car, you'll just wear out the replacement tire as well."

I'm going to teach you how to fix *yourself* by getting to the root cause behind your pain or limitation. I'll provide you with the tools you need to not only detect your own imbalances and get rebalanced, but also to quickly heal from injuries that have been nagging you for years. Before we get started, though, we must talk a little more about pain—our good friend and guide—and what it's trying to tell us.

CHAPTER 9

PAIN—YOUR GUARDIAN ANGEL

Pain has been our most reliable ally in our evolutionary bid for survival over the last six million years. Its sole function is to be a warning signal. It's a guardian angel alerting us to take our hand out of the fire, or to rest our sore knees before more damage occurs. Pain's ultimate purpose is to make sure we continue to eat, drink, sleep, procreate, and get from point A to B without damaging something crucial to our survival.

To illustrate how important pain is, the unfortunate few who don't feel pain, a condition called CIP (congenital insensitivity to pain), sadly don't often live past childhood. The reason is often because they don't get the message to withdraw from hurtful things like fire (burns are common). Other injuries and illnesses often go unnoticed because there's no way to detect there's something wrong until it's too late.

For those of us who don't have CIP, the body will always give us hints before it breaks. First, the body will whisper to us. I've heard some people refer to this whisper as a *niggle* such as a tightness in their leg or back that they didn't think much about.

If ignored, however, that *whisper* often progresses to a *yell* or a shout in the form of a strain. A strain is usually a partial muscle tear, what we might call a tweak, which is one or two steps up the pain scale from a *niggle*. Usually, we can still play through a strain, but if we still don't listen, the body will get our attention with a *scream.*

A scream comes from the type of pain we can't ignore—a pulled muscle, a herniated disc, a torn ligament, an aggravated nerve, or something else that puts us out of commission and off the tennis court.

Perhaps you can relate to this example. You run for a short ball and suddenly feel some tightness in your hamstring—a niggle. You continue playing, though, because after walking around it feels okay. Two games later, you push off that leg to get to a wide ball and you feel it again, only this time it's a little more painful. That's the *yell.*

However, you're up a break, and you think you can still take this guy (after all, you walked it off before), so you play on. Finally, your opponent hits a drop shot, and when you push off that leg to get to the ball you feel a pop.

That's the scream.

At that point you drop to the ground to get off your leg because your hamstring just tore, and now there's no ignoring or mistaking the message because you're *done.* And it was avoidable.

My advice? Don't wait for the scream.

In order to respond to the whisper or the yell before you get the scream, you first have to decipher what the pain is telling you. It's your body's way of letting you know there's an imbalance of muscular work and pressure on the joint. This means the muscle, a tendon, a ligament, or the joint itself is being overstressed.

You always get the whisper, whether you pay attention to it or not, and you usually get the yell. The shout or yell is telling you that not only is there imbalance and over-stress on your muscles or joints, but that you're on the verge of tissue damage. If you still don't listen, there could be hell to pay, and that's when you get the scream. But the scream comes too late because something is now damaged, and unless you have immediate healing powers like certain superheroes, well, tennis was fun while it lasted.

Unfortunately, we live in a culture that treats pain as if it's something to be avoided at all costs, as if pain itself is the problem. Therefore, we have all kinds of drugs, splints, multi-colored tapes, orthotics, braces, and a million other distractions and devices available that make sure we don't feel the pain or can ignore it altogether.

Unfortunately, when we deaden the body's warning system, we risk missing the message altogether, and our guardian angel's whisper may fall on deaf ears. The ensuing yell is either muffled to a whisper, or not heard at all.

You will, however, hear the scream no matter how many anti-inflammatories you take or how many braces you wear. You can't drown out the noise no matter the size of your earmuffs because the scream is the wailing siren of the arrival of an injury. Usually all you can do at that point is limp or get carried off the court.

It's important to understand that when the pain message is acknowledged early and responded to properly, you can avoid injury every time. By reading it incorrectly, such as interpreting the symptom as the cause, or by ignoring it altogether, you run the risk of real damage that can set you back for months.

When you do get the message, and we all do from time to time, the solution is to back off and restore balance.

CHAPTER 10

STATIC VS DYNAMIC STRETCHING

There's an unfortunate rumor floating in the ether that static stretching is bad or even dangerous for you, and that dynamic stretching is the only way to go. I've heard this concern from clients and athletes for years, so it's time to address the inflexible elephant in the room.

First, let's quickly define both static and dynamic stretching:

Static stretching is a comfortable muscle stretch held over a period of time, commonly between thirty seconds to two minutes, or longer. Bending over and touching your toes and holding for a minute would be an example of a static stretch (Fig. *10.1*).

Dynamic stretching occurs when you attempt to lengthen the muscles while moving a joint, or multiple joints, through a range of motion. For example, walking lunges will activate, shorten and lengthen various muscles of the hip joint during the motion with the goal of warming up and lengthening the muscles (*Fig. 10.2*).

Put simply, static stretching asks muscles to lengthen over time. Dynamic stretching asks muscles to lengthen as they move and warm up.

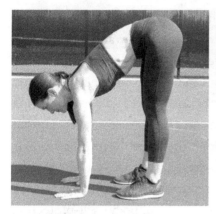

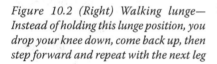

Figure 10.1 (Above) Hanging and touching your toes is an example of a static stretch

Figure 10.2 (Right) Walking lunge— Instead of holding this lunge position, you drop your knee down, come back up, then step forward and repeat with the next leg

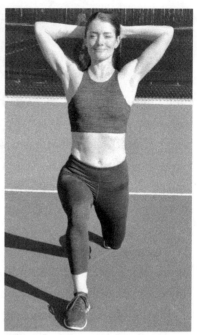

In addition to numerous studies, physical therapists, chiropractors, personal trainers, and others out there who say otherwise, and based on my twenty years of experience, saying static stretching is harmful is like saying popsicles are bad for you because you could choke on them. Aside from the occasional and extraordinarily rare occurrence, most people thoroughly enjoy them all the time without even the slightest repercussion except for a cold tongue.

As long as you're smart about how you're stretching both statically and dynamically, and you follow a few dos and don'ts, you'll be completely safe, and you'll benefit from either one.

When you do certain static stretches in this book and hold them for one, two, or even ten minutes or more, you'll feel certain muscles begin to relax over time. The muscles that are gradually letting go are the ones that have been overworking and compensating for other muscles not doing their jobs. Since muscles move bones, as the length and tension in these muscles change, the bones they attach to also change position. The results are a more neutrally positioned shoulder, pelvis, leg bone, spine, or all the above, and muscles that are balanced and functioning together again as a linked unit.

There were two reasons for all the negative hoopla over static stretching: First, people mistakenly began to associate static stretching with over-stretching, where the muscle is taken beyond its normal range of motion. In that case, when the brain detects a muscle is about to be lengthened beyond its capability, or a joint is about to be injured, it will force the muscle to reflexively shorten. This is called a *stretch reflex*, and it's an essential feature of our body's self-protection mechanism.

The fear was if the brain triggered the stretch reflex on a joint that was fixed in place during a static stretch, then the muscle would tear. However, you would never overstretch a muscle during a static stretch because you'd get the pain message way before the muscle actually tore.

To overstretch a muscle, you have to rapidly cause that muscle to lengthen, which would then trigger the brain's response to contract it. For example, getting up and sprinting to first base after sitting in a dugout for the last thirty minutes often creates hamstring pulls in baseball players because the hip joint is forced to move through a full range of motion before the muscles have had a chance to adapt to the new standing and sprinting position. It would be like getting out of a car after a long ride and sprinting to the bathroom, something you generally want to avoid.

The second reason static stretching gained a bad rap was through a few studies showing that immediately after some muscles were stretched, they produced less force than before they were stretched. For instance, if you bent down to touch your toes in order to stretch your hamstrings, those muscles would be temporarily weakened when you came up. Applied to athletes, or anyone going out for a run or a workout, that weakened condition could means a potential decrease in performance and increase in possible injury because the muscles would be less able to withstand the demand of the sport.

While those studies have merit, the next set of follow-up studies showed that even after static stretching, and even after the stretch where the muscle is now weaker, all it takes to restore its strength is to contract that muscle just a little bit. That means that after doing all the static hamstring stretches in the world, all you have to do to make sure the muscle is strong and ready for action is to bend your knee a few times to reactivate it. Problem solved.

Why does this work? Because the issue was never the muscle itself; it was the nervous system reading the position of the joint, and the length of the muscle. There are sensors in the joints and muscles that relay the joint position and muscle length back to the brain. Once the muscle was used in that new position (bending the knee to engage the hamstring), the brain/nervous system was able to recognize the new position and give it the thumbs up for full speed and strength from there.

No matter what, you can't hurt yourself while stretching if you pay attention to your body's signals. Your brain will always make sure you are aware injury is possible *before* it happens.

Never have I seen anyone hurt themselves from a stretch reflex with normal static or dynamic stretching, or with any exercise I have ever given. Nor have any of my colleagues seen anyone pull a muscle due to the stretch reflex while doing any of these exercises. *Not once, not ever.*

Don't get me wrong, it's not a myth; muscle pulls can happen with poor stretching techniques, especially if you bounce while stretching (you're taking a big chance of activating the stretch reflex). But you'll be plenty safe with any and all the exercises in this book, and with static stretching in general.

I mentioned earlier that I was a fan of dynamic and static stretching when done correctly or under the right circumstances. *Correctly* means you never push the muscle through an uncomfortable range of motion that feels more like strain than stretch.

Dynamic or static stretching under the wrong circumstances

means a few things: You're injured and shouldn't be stretching yet, or you've got to restore some symmetry to your body before going into the exercise.

Obviously, if you have a strained or pulled muscle, then you could run the risk of injuring it more by stretching before it's had time to heal.

In terms of symmetry, you want to be as balanced as possible before dynamic stretching or active motion. You want your hips and shoulders to be more level, your knees pointing straight ahead and your joints more aligned for several reasons:

1. So that there's less chance of injury.
2. So that you reinforce a positive-movement pattern and strengthen a good joint position rather than a bad one.
3. So that your body reaps the full functional benefits of the exercise in order to be ready to rock from the very first ball.

The pre-tennis routine and the *Totally Balanced Tennis Player* routine in the upcoming chapters will accomplish all three of those goals. Keep in mind as you go through the various programs and exercises that any small change to any of your joints will positively affect all the others because the body is a unit.

Wait, did I say the *body is a unit?* The body never works in pieces and parts; it always works as a unit!

CHAPTER 11

PIANO WIRE HAMMIES

recently worked with Eric, a level 5.0 player, who complained his hamstrings were always tight and touching his toes was out of the question. When he bent over to test how far he could go he reached to the middle of his shins, which was a good eight to ten inches away from his toes. Within three exercises he had his fingers on his feet. He couldn't stop shaking his head in disbelief because he hadn't touched his toes with straight legs since he was a kid.

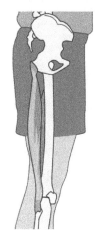

Figure 11.1

I see this excitement mixed with disbelief every day, and it can be that easy.

Let's start with how the hamstrings work. The hamstring muscles attach to bones on the bottom of your pelvis (*Fig. 11.1*).

The length and tension (and flexibility) of all muscles in your entire body are dependent on the position of the bones and joints to which they attach. Therefore, the length of the hamstrings is dependent on the position of your pelvis. If it's tucked under like you have no butt (*Fig. 11.2*), then the muscles that make up the hamstrings are in a shortened position all day long.

If your pelvis isn't tucked under, but your hip bones are forward of your ankles, that's another indicator your hamstrings are under constant tension and are probably tight (*Fig. 11.3*).

Another postural indicator of tight hamstrings is a pronounced forward rounding or extreme tightness of your upper back (*Fig. 11.4*). I don't mean Quasimodo rounding (although I'm sure his hamstrings had their issues), but a visible forward curve from below the shoulder blades up to the neck.

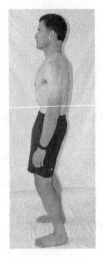 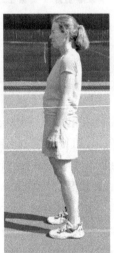 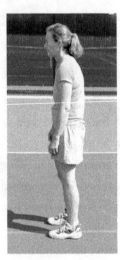

Figure 11.2 You can see there's no curve in the low back and the hips are tucked under.

Figure 11.3 Notice how the hips have swayed (moved) forward of the ankles creating constant tension on the low back.

Figure 11.4 Rounded upper back

Functionally speaking, other ways to ensure tight hamstrings are to *never* stretch, or to sit on your butt all day long. After all, we are use-it-or-lose-it creatures and we need motion to maintain motion.

Thankfully, the tightness is easily reversible for most people. Since your hamstrings attach to your pelvis, you can change the flexibility of your hamstrings in three ways:

1. Change the position of your pelvis and lower back.
2. Restore motion and a neutrally aligned position to your upper back.
3. Move more.

Why does changing your shoulders matter? Your hips are attached to the same spine as your shoulders, so you can change the *flexibility* of your hamstrings by changing the position of your shoulders.

To see and feel how this works, bend over and touch your toes. See how far you go. Now, stand with your feet pigeon-toed and interlace your fingers together. Bring your arms straight up overhead and turn your palms toward the ceiling, keeping your fingers interlaced. Pull your hands back as far as you can, tighten your thighs, keep your hips over your ankles, relax your stomach, and hold for thirty seconds (*Fig. 11.5*).

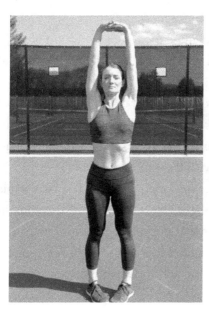

Figure 11.5 Standing Overhead Extension Feet Pigeon-Toed

The first thing you'll notice when you come out of it is that you probably feel more upright because your shoulder and upper back position have changed for the better.

Now bend over and try to touch your toes again. Many of you will notice you were able to reach further than before because your hip joint and hamstring attachments are in a different place, and your nervous system has given the joint a green light to let you bend lower. Notice that you didn't warm the hamstrings up, or stretch the hamstrings here to get more flexibility. You simply changed your alignment.

If you didn't bend any further during our little test, it means you're hopeless and have cement for hamstrings. Just kidding. It actually means the joint hasn't changed position enough yet to allow the hamstrings to let go.

Hamstrings can be stubborn. In fact, I'm sure several of you have probably noticed that you can stretch your hamstrings all day, but when you wake up the next day they're just as tight as the day before. Again, it just means you haven't changed the position of the joints the hamstrings attach to yet, and your nervous system is still tuned in to the old position.

Don't despair; you can change the range of motion of your hips and your hamstring length with a little work, and it won't take as long as you think.

In fact, much of what people consider to be hamstring inflexibility is actually due to overworked and tight back muscles which don't want to relax when you bend. The good news—it's all changeable. We'll address these issues with the exercises.

The ability to touch your toes matters when it comes to playing your best tennis and avoiding injury. Or, I should say, your spine's ability to fully bend and hips that properly rotate over your leg bone are crucial functions when bending for low volleys, reaching for any low ball, and staying down through shots without coming up early.

If your spine doesn't move properly, the risk is obvious—back strain, stress on the knees, hamstring pulls, and shoulder strain from overreaching are just a few of many possible side effects.

This hamstring routine will take about ten minutes and will restore function to your hips and length to your hamstrings. Do these exercises in exactly the order listed. Test your flexibility before and after by bending over to touch your toes.

STATIC EXTENSION
Duration: 2 minutes

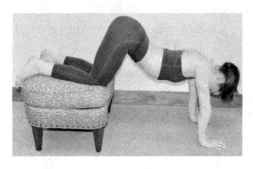

If you don't make two minutes, don't stress. This is a tough one. Begin by putting your knees on a low chair, couch, bench, or cushion. Walk your hands forward until your hips are just forward of your knees and your hands are under your shoulders. Drop your shoulder blades together as you let your chest drop toward the ground. Let your back sway and relax your stomach. Make sure to keep your arms straight, and your head dropped. Hold for two minutes. This exercise allows your hips along with your lower and upper spine to reposition into a more neutral alignment.

KNEELING GROIN STRETCH
Duration: 1 minute per side

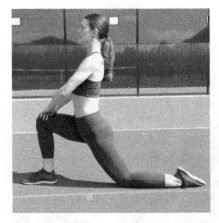

Start on your knees and step forward into a lunge position. Keep your front knee over your ankle (not in front) and let your hips sink toward the ground until you feel a stretch in the front of your trailing leg. Keep your upper body straight (don't lean forward) and relax your stomach and your shoulders.

CATS AND DOGS
Reps: 10

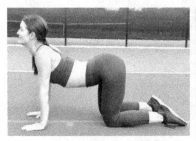 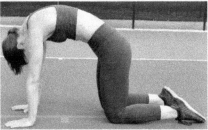

Keep your hands under your shoulders, knees under your hips, and let your back sway by initiating the motion with your hips. Let your shoulder blades drop together and look up. Next, round your back up toward the sky, roll your hips under and drop your head. Rounding your back up (cat) and down (dog) is one repetition. This exercise restores motion to your hips and spine and reminds them to work together as a unit.

DOWNWARD DOG KNEES BENT
Duration: 1 minute

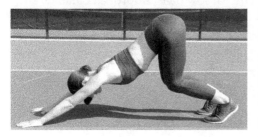

Start on your hands and knees with your hands under your shoulders and knees under your hips. Pike your hips in the air, and without moving your hands pull your hips up and back toward your heels. Pull your chest and upper body toward your knees as much as you can, keeping your knees slightly bent. This exercise restores the ability of your hips to roll forward over the femurs (upper leg bones), which is imperative in bending. The exercise also restores balanced tension between the lower spinal muscles and the muscles on the front of your hips.

AIRBENCH
Duration: 1 minute

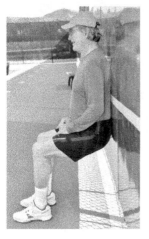

If my eighty-one-year-old dad can do it (and he's even enjoying it based on the smile on his face), so can you. Lean against a wall, walk your feet out keeping your feet straight and no wider than two fist-widths apart. Drop your hips to just above 90 degrees at the hips and knees and press your low back FLAT into the wall. There should be no space between the wall and your low back. Keep your weight toward your heels and don't forget to smile.

You can do these exercises every day and watch your hamstring and spine flexibility go from ugh to *impressive* in a very short time.

The other cool consequences of better hip and spine motion will be smoother and more efficient movement on the court, less chance of injury, increased knee bend for low balls, improved balance, and, well, winning. How's all that for motivation?

CHAPTER 12

YOUR WINNING EDGE? SYMMETRY

I f postural asymmetry is the enemy of your athletic potential, then an aligned and balanced body is its extremely benevolent fairy godmother. Therefore, the key to playing your best tennis and avoiding injury is to restore your body back to its original anatomical design. By that I mean your evolutionarily developed, genetically imprinted, completely symmetrical design.

It's your winning edge over someone less balanced and less functional, but it's also your ticket to enjoying this great sport until you're a hundred years old. Take precaution though; previously unfathomed winning bliss might also be a side effect.

Our human birthright is to be symmetrical from right to left, front to back, and top to bottom. We were born with symmetrical and level shoulders, bilaterally functioning and level hips, and identical knees and feet that point straight ahead.

Anatomical symmetry also implies that all joints and muscles are created equal, so if one joint isn't functioning optimally, or isn't identical to its counterpart, the entire musculoskeletal system is affected. Conversely, as each muscle and joint become more evenly balanced and more mobile, the entire system benefits.

Stated another way, the right side of your body should feel—and look—like the left side. The front of your body should be under equal muscle tension with the back side, and you should be able to move equally in all planes of motion.

Just like Leonardo da Vinci's geometrically proportional *Vitruvian Man,* or Michaelangelo's masterpiece *David,* we are designed to be the living picture of full, functional motion and anatomical beauty.

Let's review that perfect design:

You have eight major load joints which include both shoulders, hips, knees and ankles. We use the ear as a point of reference, too, since it sits in the middle of your head (*Fig. 12.1 and 12.2*).

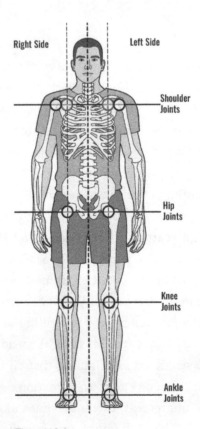

Figure 12.1

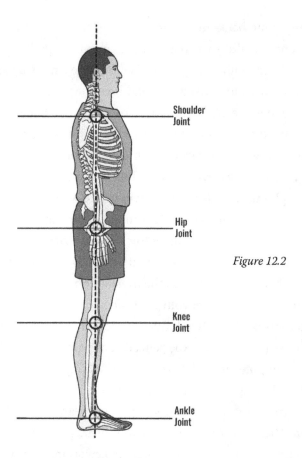

Shoulder
Joint

Hip
Joint

Figure 12.2

Knee
Joint

Ankle
Joint

Notice in the first picture *(Fig. 12.1)* showing the front of the body the shoulders, hips, knees and ankles are level with their counterparts, and the head sits directly in the middle. The right side of the body is equal and identical to the left. The two sides should also bear equal body weight.

In the second picture *(Fig. 12.2)* showing the side view, the ear lines up directly with the middle of the shoulder, hip, and knee joints, and is just barely in front of the ankle.

This is how we're designed. It's also what you'll be working to restore as you do the exercises.

The line drawn from head to toe in both pictures represents gravity as it goes through you, and it indicates where gravity is stressing your back and your joints. With your joints in perfect alignment, they absorb the force of gravity equally through the middle of each joint. They also transfer force smoothly and equally to the muscles and joints above and below.

If the line doesn't go directly through the middle of your joints, there's more stress on one part of the joint, which means some muscles are working harder than others, and there is an uneven distribution of force everywhere along the musculoskeletal chain.

The plumb line also tells us where the weight is distributed in your feet from front to back. If your shoulders and hips sit forward of that line, your weight will be toward your toes. If your shoulders sit behind the line, your weight will generally fall more toward your heels. Either way, it indicates the muscles on your front side are out of balance with those on your back side.

You probably noticed this particular front to back muscle imbalance if you've ever experienced back pain, neck pain, knee pain, or foot pain, but didn't know it had anything to do with how your joints stacked up in relation to one another.

Overall, muscle tension should be balanced in all planes of motion. Therefore, the position of your head, pelvis, spine, and major load joints tells us which muscles are overworking, or underworking, and whether those muscles are too tight, too short, or too weak.

For example, our back muscles should be under equal tension with our stomach muscles. A disruption in that tension will produce a positional change in your hips and spine.

Imagine doing sit-ups every day and thinking that if your stomach is strong, you'll be free from pain. I was one of those people. However, since muscles move bones, over-tense and engaged abdominal muscles will pull your trunk forward or tuck your butt under, taking your spine and pelvis out of their neutral alignment. The back muscles have to counterbalance that abdominal tension by tightening up; otherwise, you'd fall forward or collapse under your own weight. The result is back pain.

To give another example, over-developed chest muscles (pectoral muscles, pecs for short) round the shoulders forward and create a tug-of-war between the pecs and the upper back. The tighter your pecs from all those push-ups and bench presses, the more your upper back and shoulder joints round forward. Since your head is connected to your upper back, your head will also shift forward, straining your neck.

This brings me to the story of a sixteen-year-old boy I worked with years ago. His parents brought him in because he was complaining of shoulder pain, but they also knew something wasn't quite right about his posture. For starters, his elbows were stuck at about 45 degrees. He literally couldn't get them any straighter.

It turns out he'd been in the weight room with his friends for the last six months working on his pecs and biceps in preparation for football. He was happy to point out he could easily bench 250 pounds—just don't ask him to reach for a glass in the upper cabinet.

Aside from his bent elbows, his extreme chest and bicep tightness (the muscle on the front of arm used to bend the elbow) was pulling his shoulders and upper back forward, making him look like he was permanently hugging someone much smaller. His head and neck were also jutted forward, which meant neck pain was in his near future.

It took some time and a lot of begging from us and his parents to stay off the weights for a while. But eventually over the course of months and some hard work, he was able to get his arms (and his head) straight again.

The story has a good ending, but it highlights the merits of balanced training as well as how the body is connected. The elbow bone is connected to the shoulder bone, is connected to the back bone . . . etc.

As you can see (and maybe feel), if balanced muscle tension on any or all sides is violated, you run the risk of penalty in the form of muscle strain and pain. And frankly, that's just the tip of the iceberg. All our systems are connected, so a disruption in the balance of the musculoskeletal system can lead to problems with digestion, circulation, breathing, oxygenation of the brain and heart, and many other related symptoms too numerous to cover here.

Therefore, keeping things as balanced as possible matters. A lot.

The good news is that the closer you are to having your major load joints stack up according to your natural design, the more stress your body can handle from tennis, playing with your kids, and whatever life chooses to throw your way.

CHAPTER 13

THE FORCE IS EVERYWHERE

Most people don't realize that muscles don't just move bones. They are also major shock absorbers working to distribute force through joints. With every step we take and every ball we hit, our muscles are absorbing the force and transferring the remains to the next joint and other muscles along the chain.

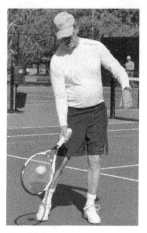

Fig. 13.1

When you hit a tennis ball, the force of hitting the ball radiates through your whole body *(Fig. 13.1)*. First, it's transferred from the strings into the racket, through the grip, and then into your wrist where the muscles of your hand and forearm absorb some of the shock and transfer the rest into the elbow joint.

It goes from there into the muscles of your upper arm and shoulder, where it's dispersed into your upper back. Every step of the way, the muscles are absorbing as much force as they can and then transferring

75

the remainder to the next joint and its surrounding muscles and connective tissue (fascia, tendons, ligaments).

If that force transmission and absorption is disrupted *anywhere* along the way, then it gets transferred to some muscles and tissues more than others, or some parts of the joint more than others, and those parts either wear away faster than normal or become injured.

How does it get disrupted? Anywhere a joint is out of position due to traumatic injury or imbalanced muscles.

My father's body is a good example. In college, he suffered a major left knee injury playing football. Back in the 1950s they didn't have the medical knowledge we do today, so they pieced it back together the best they could, but his knee was never the same. Even after therapy, his left knee never recovered its full weight-bearing capacity. In fact, it was never able to fully straighten again. As a result, he shifted more of his weight to his right knee and right hip to compensate, and his right hip joint was the first to be replaced many years later.

He's a total gamer, though. He was back speed skating a few weeks after his hip surgery, and at eighty-plus years he's playing tennis and still working out several days a week. He's doing his functional exercises every day now because he wants to continue to play until he's one hundred.

Hopefully by now you're starting to get the picture. When the position of any joint is compromised, the function of that joint is compromised. It then becomes vulnerable to injury or pain, *and* so do the joints above and below.

My goal is to help you avoid any joint replacements and pain. If you're already on that unfortunate path and stuck in the mud, the next task is to give you the tools to dig yourself out.

In the meantime, your postural and mechanical imbalances have been hiding in plain sight, and it's time to put them in the spotlight.

PART III

ASSESS TO PROGRESS

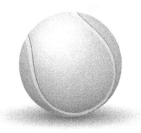

CHAPTER 14

YOUR BEAUTIFUL SELF
. . . ASSESSMENT

I t's time to identify the imbalances in your muscles, bones and
joints. We'll call them postural imbalances for short. They matter
because you'll have to adapt your movement or your stroke
mechanics to accommodate and compensate for these imbalances,
and your game and your body will suffer.

The consequences include wasting energy, poor stroke technique,
guaranteed physical limitation, eventual pain and injury, and not
reaching anywhere near your tennis potential.

This section may be the most important in the entire book because
the questions herein are designed to get you in touch with your own
body. You can then use that information to learn how to fix yourself.

Understanding and owning your own habits, challenges,
and limitations is also the first step down the path to taking full
responsibility for your health, healing and preventing injuries,
improving your game, playing without limitation, and enjoying this
game for as long as possible.

What you're about to discover will not only be illuminating, it
will be extremely motivating. When most people see and feel their

own postural imbalances, they're usually shocked and motivated into taking immediate action.

First, take off your shoes. They're an impediment to your brain sensing your position in space, and they get in the way of your body awareness. Once they're off, find a comfortable stance and close your eyes (after reading this paragraph, that is). Notice where your weight distribution is in your feet.

Does it feel like there is more pressure or weight on one foot than the other?

Is the weight on the inside or outside of your feet?

Is there more weight toward your toes or toward your heels?

Really try to feel it. You may notice your feet feel completely different from one another. There might be more weight on the inside front of one foot, and toward the back and the outside of the other.

You might feel much more weight in one foot compared to the other, or maybe you can't quite tell which side is carrying more of your weight. There are no right or wrong answers here. The point is for you to feel it and get in touch with your own body because no matter what you discover now, it's going to feel different and more balanced once you begin to do the exercises.

Now that you have an idea of where your weight distribution is, look at your feet.

Are they turned out?

Is one foot more turned out than the other?

Is one foot slightly ahead of the other (a sign of hip rotation)?

Now find a mirror and look at your shoulders.

Are your shoulders level?

It's very common to see one shoulder lower than the other in many people, but especially in tennis players (a sign of shoulder blade and back muscle imbalance).

When you look at your hands in the mirror is one hand in front of the other?

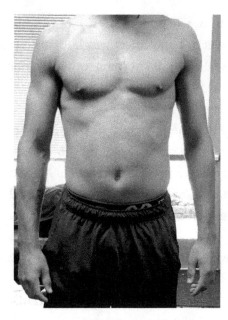

Figure 14.2 Look at where the right hand is sitting compared to the left. This is a common sign of trunk rotation.

Do you see the backs of both hands, or one hand and not the other?

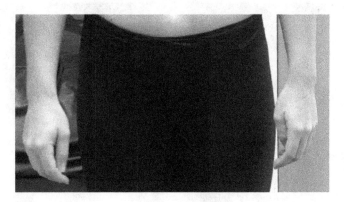

Figure 14.3 You can clearly see the back of both hands rather than just the thumb and forefinger.

Your hand position is indicative of your shoulder position, as well as the amount of internal rotation of your arm bone. When looking in the mirror, you should only see your thumb and pointer finger, rather than the backs of your hands.

Is your head straight or does it look like it's slightly listing to one side?

Our heads weigh ten to twelve pounds, so if your head is even slightly off to one side, it will not only affect weight distribution in your hips and feet, but it will also put enormous strain on one side of the muscles and vertebrae of your neck.

How about your hips. Do they look level?

If you can't tell by looking, then put each of your hands on top of your hip bones. You should be able to see if they look level, or if one is higher than the other. An *elevated hip* is a sign of hip rotation, uneven weight distribution, imbalanced hip muscles, imbalanced back muscles, and a host of other things. Don't worry, though; you'll *easily* fix this.

Now look at your kneecaps. Where does each knee point? Does it point in, or out, or does it look like it's pointing straight ahead?

Sometimes this is difficult to see, so more importantly, ask yourself: *Do your knees look the same or different?*

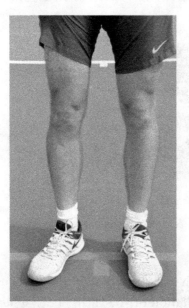 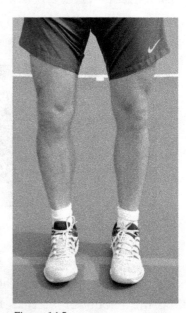

Figure 14.4   *Figure 14.5*

In the first pic (*Fig. 14.4*) you can see the right knee clearly pointing in with relation to the foot and you can see both kneecaps are pointing in very different directions. In the second figure (*Fig. 14.5*) you can see both kneecaps clearly pointing out in relation to the feet.

Knees that point out can be a sign of glute and hip flexor tightness. Knees that point in are a sign of imbalanced hip flexors with the lower back muscles, tight lateral hips, and potential shoulder rounding among other things.

I use the phrase "among other things" because every imbalance indicates a host of other imbalances all over the body. The body is a unit. Everything is literally connected via connective tissue, but also through gravity. You can't turn a knee out without affecting the foot. You can't turn a foot out without rotating the hips, and you can't rotate the hips without affecting the shoulders. If one shoulder drops down, the opposite side of the body has to work against gravity to counterbalance it.

Feel it for yourself. Turn out one foot to 45 degrees and notice what your knee does. Where did your hips go? What did your opposite arm or shoulder do?

Now you can understand that if you treat knee pain with exercises that just strengthen the muscles around the knee, you're probably missing the rest of the picture, and the point. In order to truly fix that knee, you might have to address the misaligned shoulder position, which takes the hip out of rotation, which in turn automatically realigns and rebalances the knee joint and the muscles around it. And you didn't have to do a thing to strengthen the knee.

So far, we've been focused on determining where your major load joints (shoulders, hips, knees and ankles) are positioned, and they're helping you to determine imbalances in weight distribution, joint overload, and muscle tension.

Now look at your muscles.

Look at your chest (pec) muscles. Do they look the same? How about your calf muscles?

Very often in tennis players one calf is slightly bigger than the other.

Look at your abs.

Is one side more defined?

Again, this is another sign of upper body rotation, and muscle imbalance all the way down the muscle chain to your foot and up to your neck.

It will be extremely helpful to write down what you found because it's going to change, and it's easy to forget what you started with. Keeping a record of where you started will help you see where you've been and how much you've evolved and progressed along the way. This improvement is not only fulfilling and awesome, but it will give you motivation to continue to balance out your body and then to maintain it.

Take Pictures

Another record I suggest you keep is a photo of yourself. We take postural pictures of everyone in the clinic so they can see their imbalances, and then we take them again after a week or a few weeks of doing the exercises so they can see how much they've changed.

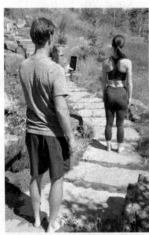

Have someone close to you take photos of you from head to toe from your front, back, and both sides wearing just shorts if you're a guy, or shorts and a sports bra if you're a woman. No shoes. Don't think about how to stand, don't try to stand up straight, etc. Just be. And try to stand just like you would if you weren't thinking about your posture *(Fig. 14.6)*.

Now print out your photos, and on the front and back-view pictures draw a line from the middle of your feet straight up to your head. This divides your body into right and left halves.

Figure 14.6 Taking posture pics

Look at your feet, knees, shoulders, and head again and discover for yourself what you see. Are you listed to one side? Is one shoulder higher or lower? Does one foot point out more than the other? What you see might shock you, but don't worry. This is only the starting point.

Next, use the side-view pictures to draw a line with your pen and ruler from the front of your ankle bone straight up to the top of the page. Keep the line perfectly vertical. Now look where your ear is in relation to your shoulder.

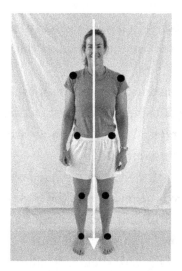

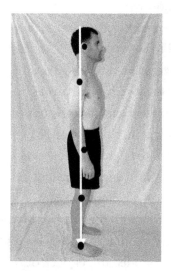

Figure 14.7 Draw a line from the middle of the feet straight up on the front view.

Figure 14.8 Draw a line from just barely in front of the ankle joint straight up to see where your major load joints are positioned in relation to each other.

Is your head forward?

Put a dot on your hip joint, which will be just above the middle of your butt if you are looking at it from the side. Add another dot on the middle of your knee, and one more on the middle of your shoulder joint.

Do the dots line up?

The side-view pictures are perfect for seeing how your major load joints stack up and where the pressure is on your spine from your neck to your low back.

You've seen in the previous chapter how your major load joints should ideally stack up. Now, by looking at these pictures, you can easily see if your upper back and shoulders are rounding, if your head is forward of your shoulders, if one foot is in front of the other, if your hips are forward of your knees and ankles, and other imbalances. Whatever you do, don't judge yourself. Everyone has some imbalances, and most people have many, so you're in very good company.

Remember, *everything you see is fixable*, but it's important to see it and to begin to understand how these postural imbalances you've discovered are affecting you.

A forward head indicates there is too much stress on the muscles of your head and neck and upper back. This stress could present itself as neck pain, headaches, TMJ, nerve referral going down your arm, or even just tight shoulder and neck muscles.

Forward hips represent strain on the muscles of your lower back, and a general imbalance between the muscles on the front of your body with the muscles on the back of your body. Rounded and forward shoulders almost always follow forward swayed hips.

A rounded upper back or rounded forward shoulders indicates shoulder muscle imbalance and dysfunction, as well as strain on the lower back, tension in the mid back, and stress on your neck.

Aside from the pictures, another great test to check your head position and your posture is to stand with your heels, butt, and shoulders (relaxed, not pulled back) against a wall.

When you put your head on the wall does it feel relaxed and normal, or do you have to tilt your chin up and reach your head back to get it to the wall?

Are your eyes still level or does it seem as if you're looking up?

Obviously, if you can't get your head on the wall at all, that speaks volumes. That scenario is common, though, and indicates a very rounded and tight upper back. It also indicates an imbalance in the muscles of the hips, knees and ankles because if the upper back is rounded forward, the entire muscular chain is disrupted from head to toe.

If you feel like you're about to fall forward, that's a sign your body is used to pitching forward and catching itself with your overworked calf, hamstring and lower back muscles. Obviously, you'll feel an exaggerated arch in your low back. Let it happen.

This isn't really how your lower back would feel under perfectly aligned posture, but standing against the wall allows your head, shoulders, hips, knees and ankles to stack up as they should, which gives you an idea of what it feels like to be perfectly straight. Or in many cases, it will remind you that you're, well, not.

CHAPTER 15

READY FOR THE CIRCUS? YOUR FUNCTIONAL TESTS

Now that you've explored your postural imbalances, let's dive into the function of your joints and muscles. Your posture provides a snapshot of your joint function. A forward head is not only a sign the muscles of your head and neck are working too hard, but it's also a sign the range of motion in your neck may be compromised. An arm bone that's rotated in is an indication that the shoulder joint isn't gliding smoothly and you're lacking power on your serve.

Every joint is designed for a full range of motion and stability to allow us to bend, twist, reach, push, pull, jump, somersault, back flip, dive for volleys, slap forehand winners on the run, and serve anywhere from 30 to 130 mph. If there's any question of what our amazing bodies are capable of, go to a Cirque Du Soleil show. What these performers can do is a dazzling display of what's humanly possible.

I'm not saying we can all be contortionists, but I am saying that we were born with the ability to back handspring across the room, walk on our hands, swing from bars set fifty feet off the ground, and fold in half from our hips, among other feats of athletic amazingness.

Most of us don't or can't do these things because we never trained to do it from a young age. Yet, we *could* have, and we can still restore some or much of that function because that's what our bodies—all our bodies—are designed to do.

Again, I'm not saying that after twenty years of not touching your toes you'll be doing the splits soon, although I do believe even that's possible with enough focus and hard work. What I am saying is that by doing some simple things you can remind the body of what it *is* capable of, and you can make massive improvements given the desire and the right stimulus.

Each exercise that follows is a simple functional test that isolates a joint on your spine. I chose these exercises for their simplicity and your ability to do them on your own. They don't require precise measurements or scientific analysis, just your eyes and your kinesthetic sense.

You've already tested some of your spinal motion by touching your toes in the chapter on tight hamstrings, so let's begin by checking out your spinal rotation.

Your spine's ability to rotate fully from bottom to top is crucial to keeping you free from injury and on the tennis court.

Aside from potential for injury, turning to hit a forehand, backhand, or serve without being able to maximally rotate will lead to less power, more strain, and a search for a better racket to compensate for all of the above.

This exercise is called the *Upper Spinal Floor Twist*. We use it in our clinics all the time to restore motion and flexibility to all parts of the spine. You'll use it now as a starting point to test the rotational function of your spine. You can watch a video of each of these upcoming functional tests at www.egoscue.com/agelesstennis.

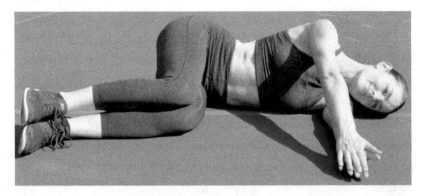

Figure 15.1 The Upper Spinal Floor Twist

Start off by lying on your side with your knees and hips at 90 degrees and stacked perfectly on top one another (*Fig. 15.1 above*). Keeping your knees together, rotate your top arm over to the other side with your palm up facing the ceiling (*Fig. 15.2*). Turn your head toward your open hand and let your hand drop as far as it can toward the ground, keeping your arm straight out from your shoulder. Don't let your top knee slide off the bottom knee even a little to make sure the rotation comes from your mid and upper back rather than your hips.

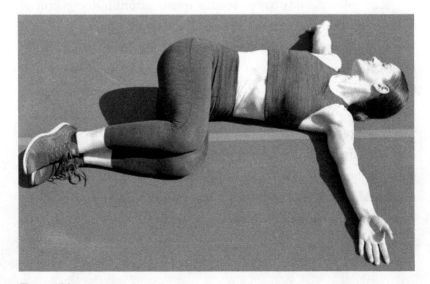

Figure 15.2

The test is to see how much of your arm rests on the ground. If the back of your hand and most of your arm are touching the ground while keeping your knees perfectly stacked, then you have good rotation. If your hand or arm don't touch the ground at all, or just the fingertips touch, then you have some work to do.

Next, we'll do two tests for your hips. The first exercise will test the amount of external rotation of your hip joint and the next your internal rotation. Both hip functions are required to keep your hips from injury as well as your knees and ankles. If the hip joints don't properly rotate, then your low back and your knees will be the first to compensate, which puts them in the line of fire.

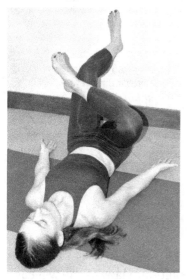

This exercise is called the *Assisted Hip Lift* (*Fig. 15.3*). It isolates one hip at a time to measure the amount of external rotation in the joint. Start by lying on your back with your feet up on the wall and your knees bent at 90 degrees. Cross your right ankle over your left knee and use your right leg muscles to push your knee toward the wall. Make sure your right ankle isn't doing the moving by keeping that ankle joint on your knee rather than just your foot.

Figure 15.3 Assisted Hip Lift Test

The test is to see how far your knee can get toward the wall without shifting your opposite hip to help. Your right knee should be at least parallel to the wall. Anything short of that indicates some limitation in the motion of your hip joint.

The even more interesting comparison will be between your left and right sides. When you test the left hip try to notice if it's different from the right. It likely will be for many people, and that's okay for now. Keep in mind, this is all just a starting point.

The test for internal rotation is called the *Wishbone.* You might have to do this in front of a mirror or have someone take a picture of you so you can see your feet. Lie on your stomach and bend your knees to 90 degrees so the bottoms of your feet point up toward the ceiling. Touch your knees together and let your feet fall out away from each other. The test is to see how far they fall and how alike they are. Obviously, you'll need to be lying in front of a mirror to see your feet, or have your friend or partner take a picture.

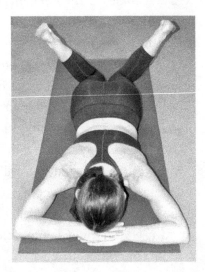

Figure 15.3 Wishbone for the internal rotation of your hip joint

Your feet and lower legs should be at least a 45-degree angle to the floor to signify a good amount of rotation. Many of you will have more, some will have much less, especially on one side. If you notice a limitation or a big discrepancy, make sure you repeat this test after several days or weeks of doing the exercises.

The final exercise will test both your shoulders and upper back (*Fig. 15.4*). Lie down on your back with your legs up on a couch or chair and your knees bent to 90 degrees. You can also use a wall for this by putting your feet on a wall with your hips and knees at 90 degrees. Now bring your elbows out to your sides so they're on the ground but level with your shoulders. Next, point your fingers up toward the ceiling and then let the back of your hands drop toward the ground above your head. This is the put-em-up position, only you're on your back with the back of your hands on the ground rather than standing with an outlaw pointing a gun at you.

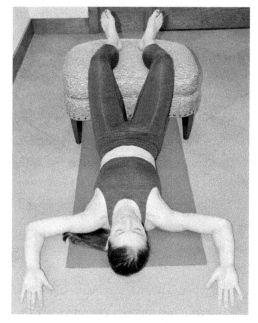

Figure 15.4 Arm glide position

Your wrists and the back of both hands should be easily and completely on the ground if your shoulders are functioning correctly and symmetrically. However, you might notice that one hand didn't drop as far as the other, or one wrist just isn't close to touching the floor.

If this is the case, you're in good company. I'd say eight out of ten people who walk through my clinic door can't get both hands on the ground equally, and four out of those eight can't get one hand, or either, on the ground.

This is a great test of shoulder function as well as a test for rounding (flexion) of your upper back. It's also another test of your head position. If you can't get your head on the ground comfortably without putting something behind it like a pillow, or if it feels like you have to look back to get your head on the ground, then your neck is under strain while standing, too.

Definitely try this position again immediately after doing your exercises, and then again in one to two weeks. You'll be amazed at how quickly your shoulder function and upper back position can change, but you have to put in the work.

Even a small amount of shoulder dysfunction can have a big impact on the rest of your body since your wrist, elbow, rotator cuff muscles, and your lower back will have to compensate for shoulders that aren't functioning correctly. If you're experiencing pain in any of these areas, then this lack of shoulder function, and/or a rounded and tight upper back is likely the cause, or are at least significantly contributing to the problem.

It goes without saying that serving, rotating, hitting an overhead, and every other shot in tennis requires good shoulder and upper back function. Therefore, restoring it will make an enormous impact on your game and on your life.

Speaking of life, these tests are given within the context of tennis, but they're also indicative of how much function you have off the court. Every exercise you do, every movement you make, every tennis shot and golf ball you hit is a functional test. I'll give you the upcoming exercises to help your tennis game, but in truth, they'll do much more.

They'll affect every aspect of your daily life; picking up your daughter should get easier, gardening will be less stress on your back, standing for long periods of time won't bother you so much. You might hit a PR in the weight room or find that even reaching in the backseat to get your jacket no longer strains your arm. It's exciting to imagine how much your game can improve, but it will be equally exciting to observe how much easier the functional demands of your life will become.

CHAPTER 16

THE ORIGINS OF YOUR IMBALANCE

At this point you're probably wondering where all these imbalances came from. It's an important question considering there might be something you can do outside these exercises to reinforce a positive change or to eliminate anything contributing to the problem.

Let's begin with the simple fact that tennis is a very one-sided sport. It's much less one-sided than golf or baseball, which ask for rotation only in one direction. But in tennis we still use one arm and one side of the body more than the other.

The way we play can also make a difference. Some players hit 60 percent to 70 percent more forehands than backhands in a match—especially the pros. They run around their backhands to crank forehands in order to open the court and to dictate the point.

If you're right handed and a high level player, most forehands are now hit with an open stance and the majority of the work and stress falls on the right hip. If you're not a pro and have a more traditional style of play, most of the work is focused on the left hip from landing on the left foot while serving and from transferring your weight to the left leg during a forehand.

The imbalanced workload between hips would be like lifting weights with a twenty-pound weight in one hand, and a ten-pound weight in the other for hours on end. When it comes time to stretch your arms, it's easy to guess which one would be tighter, much more fatigued, and more vulnerable to injury.

Incidentally, 99 percent of the time the side that's bearing more weight or doing more work is almost always the first to break down. The muscles, tendons, and joints on that side simply can't endure the strain over a long period of time.

Past injuries are also common instigators of muscular, mechanical, and postural imbalances over time. Let's say you tore your left ACL playing soccer or skiing some years ago, and your body sensed the injury and brilliantly compensated by putting more of your weight on the non-injured side.

Even after returning to 100 percent, our bodies often fail to transfer the weight completely back on that formerly injured side. You can often see it or feel it while walking or running in the form of a slight limp or a continued hitch in your giddy-up. The reason is our nervous systems learn to integrate a new compensating pattern of standing and moving as a result of major injury.

I know what you're thinking: *Can't I just strengthen the side that's underworking with one-sided exercises?* Yes, you can, and that will absolutely improve the strength and stability on that side. However, until you train your body and your nervous system to work together as a unit again (shoulders, hips, knees and ankles reconnecting), one-sided strengthening won't be enough.

Why? The body doesn't work in pieces and parts, and anyone who treats it that way is treating the symptom and missing the bigger picture. I've also been working with post-rehab injuries for twenty years, and most of the time—even after rehab—most people still don't equally use both sides. The disparity is always noticeable in their gait, and especially evident when playing sports.

Aside from one-sided sports and injuries, additional sources for imbalance can be bad habits. For instance, women should never wear their purse on the same shoulder because it will throw their shoulders and back muscles off. Guys should avoid sitting on a wallet in their back pocket every day because it throws off the alignment of their hips and spine. New parents should avoid carrying their children on one hip all the time because it can also shift their hips out of whack and lead to back problems.

You might ask if handedness plays a role. It does, but only when you're asked to do repetitive things with that hand for months or years like hammering, or some other task that requires the use of one arm or hand (or leg, for that matter) repeatedly like you would in tennis. Otherwise, handedness doesn't have to make a meaningful difference, especially once you're doing exercises that counterbalance it.

Your job can also play a role. I stopped counting how many dentists I see in my clinic every month. Their job requires them to sit or stand in a twisted position for hours every day. Their stressed and often twisted frames hobble in with back pain, or a neck strain, or a disc herniation, and they're worried their job and career is in jeopardy. Once we help them get untwisted and out of pain, we give them daily exercises to counteract the rotation and postural strain they suffer.

Of course, not all dentists are twisted up, and there are many other professions that routinely foster imbalance. In terms of your profession, ask yourself these questions:

1. Does my job ask me to repeat a certain skill with one side of my body over many hours, days, weeks, or months?
2. Do I have to sit through much of the day?
3. Do I sit with one leg always crossed over the other?
4. Do I have to stand for my work, and if so, do I have to twist to the same side all the time?

I heard the story of one of our clients who, as mayor of the city, had to reach for his phone across his desk all day. And it rang a lot. When he couldn't understand why the exercises weren't working, the therapist asked to observe the man at work.

It became clear within minutes that his right low back was bothering him because his phone was way too far away and always on the right side. The man was reaching for his phone all day, almost like doing the same stretch on the same side over and over and over again without ever doing the other side. Once the therapist moved his phone directly in front of him, and within a short reach, the pain abated. It can be as easy as that with you, too.

I encourage you to begin to pay attention to all your work and home habits that have so far been unconscious. How do you stand when you cook, do the dishes, brush your teeth? How do you sit when you're on the couch or in your favorite chair? When you're standing around what leg do you stand on? You might be amazed at what you discover and how it relates to any pain or imbalance you're carrying around.

By the way, get rid of any mattresses you own that are over ten years old or have developed well-worn troughs. A wavy, bumpy mattress doesn't do you any good no matter how perfect your posture. It doesn't matter if the new mattress is hard or soft, just pick one that's comfortable.

I was the victim of an old and decrepit mattress several years ago. My wife had left town, so I took over the entire bed like a happy pet enjoying the cushy comfort and space even though the mattress didn't feel even. I realized as I spread out that the two of us had molded two troughs on the sides of the mattress where we normally slept with a big lumpy bump in the middle between us. It didn't deter me, though, because after all, I had the whole bed to myself! The next morning at work I noticed a nagging pain on one side of my back and it didn't go away for three days.

I finally decided to sleep back on my side in my worn trough. It turned out that sleeping in the middle of that uneven mattress was throwing a big rotation into my hips and back (surprise, surprise). Once I went back to my groove, the pain immediately ceased and never returned.

Then I got a new mattress.

CHAPTER 17

THE TRUTH ABOUT WEIGHTLIFTING

The topic of weight training can be a touchy subject because we live in a fitness-obsessed culture that often sends the message that we must lift weights and frequent the gym to be healthy and strong. But what kind of strength do we really need to be healthy or to be a better athlete?

Despite the potential to upset a few diehards (sorry, Arnold), gym attendance and health don't always go hand in hand and sometimes weight training can be as hurtful as it can be helpful. Bad form and technique, using the same machines and weights all the time, and added demand to crooked and imbalanced bodies showing up to get their pump on are just a few reasons.

Don't get me wrong, I'm not against weights. When you begin lifting with a more functional, balanced and symmetrical frame they'll add tremendous strength, challenge, and enjoyment to your exercise routine. In fact, regardless of your current condition, weights can be very beneficial for anyone when done correctly, and strength training can be tremendously helpful with the right guidance and mindset. So, I'll do my best to illuminate a path you can easily follow.

There's a big difference between weight training and functional strength training. You can functionally strength train with weights, but you don't always get functional strength just by using weights. By functional strength, I mean strength that actually translates to your sport and makes you better at it, especially strength that transfers to tennis. More importantly, the wrong kind of either training can injure you, and almost always does.

With athletes or anyone else entering the gym, the first problem is the imbalanced body showing up to weight train. The second problem is the mindset and assumption that getting stronger is better. The final issue, particularly for athletes, is the common practice of increasing the weight and/or the volume of training without regard to the athlete's particular sport, position, or individual imbalances. Together, these practices often result in an individual or athlete who's overworked and injured, more imbalanced, or less flexible, or all the above.

Unfortunately, gyms are often breeding grounds for dysfunctional training partly because people typically train the vanity muscles, or *peacock* muscles. Like peacocks who brandish their beautiful feathers to find mates, these are the muscles we flex while naked in the mirror hoping our partners will be so impressed they'll be overtaken with desire. Thus, the pecs, abs, and biceps get the bulk of attention for many of us guys, while the glutes, hamstrings and abs often get the bulk of attention from many of the gals.

Most people also don't know what to do in the gym (understandably), so they usually stick to the exercises they know. The problem is, they end up using the same machines and repeating the same exercises all the time, which leads to the same muscles being worked every time they visit the gym. Welcome to the world of imbalanced strength and muscle development.

Our muscles, our joints and nervous systems demand *varied* motion and stimulus to maintain function as well as balance. Remember, we adapt to the stimulus we give ourselves. Sitting over long periods of time leads to tight hips, rounded backs, forward heads and lazy postural muscles. Weight training leads to stronger and bigger muscles.

Therefore, how we sit, and how we train makes all the difference in how our bodies adapt and respond. The next time you head to the gym, use all the machines or try to vary your exercises to stimulate as many muscles and body parts as possible.

Avoid thinking, *Today is chest and back day, and tomorrow is legs and biceps day.* Instead think, *Today is whole body day, and so is tomorrow, and the next day, and the next.*

The mantra among *Egoscue* therapists is, *Straighten before you strengthen.* Get the body balanced (or as balanced as possible) before going into the weight room so you strengthen a good posture and a good joint position, rather than reinforce an imbalanced or a bad joint position.

Nine times out of ten, the tennis player, football player or average Jane who goes into the weight room with a rotated hip and a shoulder imbalance is coming out of the weight room with an even more rotated hip, and an even bigger shoulder imbalance. The reason is that our bodies run away from our weakest points and toward our strongest points under demand. The more the demand, the more the imbalance will show up.

Put simply, the bigger the weights, the more your body has to compensate, and the more imbalanced you get. The more imbalanced you get, the worse your performance, and the bigger the chance of injury. It happens every single day in every gym and weight room in the country.

Every personal trainer, strength trainer, or physical therapist has had to correct someone's form in a lunge or a squat because they were listing to one side as they lowered, or a knee was collapsing in, or they rotated too much one way. However, the bad form wasn't a result of the exercise; it's a result of a dysfunctional body going into the exercise. And most people don't have trainers watching over them when they lift.

Countless other form *faux pas* often go unnoticed but not unpunished. In fact, the postural form violations I see every day in the weight room are numerous and unending, and unfortunately so are the nagging pains and injuries they cultivate.

I don't include a specific weight routine because it's my belief that with the functional strength routines, you'll get everything you need—and more. Plus, there are plenty of books out there on weight training already without me adding to the clutter.

However, I recognize that many enjoy lifting for the way it makes them feel and for the noticeable strength gains. I'm one of those people. There is absolutely no question that weightlifting will make you stronger, and it can help your game under the right circumstances, but remember you also want functional strength to go with it. These tips will help you accomplish that goal, and they will give you some very specific things to focus on while lifting in order to make sure you're getting the most out of your workout while decreasing your chance of injury now and later.

The most important piece of advice and overall theme to these tips is to train and strengthen good posture at all times, as opposed to training a poor one. Remember, you always want to train your nervous system through a positive reinforcement pattern, not one that could be detrimental to your posture or to your joint health.

To that end, here are my tips for lifting weights:

1. Always train with your feet pointing straight ahead no matter what position you're in—sitting, standing or lying. You want to train your body to be equal and balanced, so your feet should always be equal and balanced when lifting.

2. Your shoulder blades should be squeezed together as much as possible for any shoulder or arm exercises, and just about any weight exercise you do while sitting or standing *(Fig. 17.1)*. Keeping your shoulder blades

together when possible will help strengthen your posture, and it will ensure you're getting bilateral (even) demand from right to left, as opposed to working different muscles on each side and creating an imbalance. For instance, if you're doing bicep curls, do them with your heels, hips, and head against a wall with your shoulder blades squeezed together while lifting. If you're doing bench presses, keep your shoulder blades squeezed together the entire time as you would when doing a functional push-up.

3. If you find yourself having to round your upper back forward to lift a weight, then use a lighter weight or change the exercise altogether.

4. Vary your training as much as possible. As I said earlier, use many different machines, train as many different muscles together, and vary the exercises you do even if they seem to work the same muscles. For example, if you're doing triceps exercises, do triceps dips one day, overhead triceps extensions another day, and triceps pulldowns another. All these exercises hit the triceps, but they're all different enough to stimulate the nervous system's need for variety, and they work many different muscles in addition to the triceps.

5. Roll your hips forward to create an arch in your low back in all sitting exercises (*Fig. 17.3*). When your feet are straight, your shoulder blades are squeezed together, and your hips are rolled forward, you are now training a balanced posture from right to left, all the core stabilizers will be engaged, and your whole body will be working together as a unit.

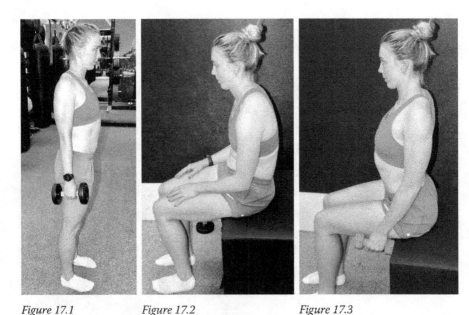

Figure 17.1   *Figure 17.2*   *Figure 17.3*

Figure 17.1 showing the shoulder blades squeezed back, and feet straight while lifting weights. Figures 17.2 and 17.3 showing the incorrect way to sit while lifting followed by the correct way with hips rolled forward, feet straight and shoulder blades squeezed.

6. Always train your muscles through a full range of motion. I see too many people doing biceps curls without going to full elbow extension or full flexion, or I see them doing push-ups and only going partway down. If you can't do the full range of motion, then you're holding too much weight. So, you might have to decrease the reps, or you might have to decrease the weight to get the job done correctly.

7. Never compromise form to lift more weight. If you have to rock, or sway back and forth to get the weight up, it's too much weight.

8. Never, never, never push through pain. Strength training of any kind is only as good for you as it feels. If it doesn't feel good, or right, then stop. Trust me, it can do more harm than good if you ignore the pain.

9. Never compromise your flexibility and function for strength. If you begin to notice a decrease in the amount of flexibility in your neck, back, shoulders, hips, hamstrings, or anywhere else from lifting weights or strength training, then it's time to back off, restore your flexibility back to where it was before, and adjust your training techniques, even if that just means adding a post-weight rebalancing routine to restore postural balance and functional mobility. Remember, mobility and stability always trump strength. In fact, mobility and stability beget strength, not the other way around.

10. If you always remember to strengthen your body, not your ego, you'll be sure to stay out of trouble. Lift less weight or do fewer reps if it means maintaining your form. Form first, ego never.

Keep in mind, your health is not measured by how many miles you can run, how much weight you can lift, how many push-ups and sit-ups you can do, or by how many times a week you visit the gym.

Your health is determined by how willing and able you are to respond to your needs physically, mentally, and emotionally, how much vitality and energy you have, and most of all, how much you're enjoying on a daily basis this experience we call life. Let happiness be your gauge of overall wellness.

CHAPTER 18

INJURIES AND ATHLETES UNDER SIEGE

Andy Murray is one of the fastest and most talented tennis players of our era. However, from my observation (and I've never met Andy) he had been majorly overtraining in 2016 and 2017. The evidence was in his posture. He looked *yoked*, which is great for the beach, but not necessarily beneficial for a productive year of tennis, as he found out. Yoked muscles can sometimes lead to tight muscles, which is how he appeared to me.

His abs and pecs were way too *tonic*, which is another way of saying overly engaged to the detriment of his other muscles. Also, his upper body leaned too far forward in relation to his hips. That indicated to me that he had very tight hip flexors, which along with the vertical force of gravity, can lead to tremendous stress on the lower back and compromise the diaphragm function, making it tough to breathe and recover after long points.

So right off the bat, I could see he had a tighter than normal upper body, a tight lower body, and a low back that wasn't very mobile or bearing weight evenly. Obviously, none of those issues are conducive to feeling good or playing well.

Back pain was inevitable with all that going on, but the straw that broke this formidable player's muscle-bound back was his right to left imbalance. Murray was overloading his right hip, which created a constant over-stress on that ankle, knee and hip joint.

It was especially evident in one of his last matches; he walked back to get a ball at one point, and I noticed his entire pelvis rotate as his right leg went back behind him. A pelvis with fully functioning and mobile hip joints doesn't do that.

When the hip joint stops rotating and moving independently of the pelvis, you're in big trouble. The result for Murray was a right hip injury, which resulted in several surgeries culminating in a total hip replacement.

Could he have avoided it? We'll never know, and it doesn't matter now. What does matter is the signs of musculoskeletal dysfunction and impending injury were right there for all to see, as they almost always are. The key is to recognize the signs and catch it early. The reason you're reading this book is to avoid potential injuries or to banish those you have.

As for Murray, thankfully for all of us fans he has returned to playing doubles and is even gracing the singles court once again. He's a fighter and a true champion who has become a beacon of hope for anyone dreaming of competing at a high level with a former major injury and especially a prosthetic hip!

I hope from here on out he adjusts his training and his mindset to recognize that just being stronger doesn't necessarily mean better. Athletes need balanced strength along with full mobility, especially when there are large imbalances present. If not, diminished performance and injury won't be far behind.

Murray isn't the only top athlete who's battled with injury though. Every year male and female athletes of every sport become injured to the point of having to take months off. Many have lost major time along with numerous opportunities to further their legacies. For me, it's very sad but not surprising given the imbalances that they clearly—and unknowingly—train and compete with. Yet, it's my belief they're all fixable.

And so are you!

How many times over the years have you had to forgo playing due to an injury? Thousands of recreational players around the globe are commonly forced to sit on the sideline for days, weeks, or months as they struggle to heal from acute or chronic injuries and pain. Your goal is to diminish the frequency, the healing time and the overall number and severity of injuries you suffer throughout your playing days and your life.

Of course, injury happens to everyone at some time or other no matter how well you train, especially when you consider that many injuries have an emotional root, not just physical.

However, they can happen a lot less frequently for anyone, especially you, as you develop a more kinesthetic awareness of your body, an improved understanding of how posture and joint position relates to injury, and commit to some more targeted work toward balancing your body going into training, and before going on the tennis court.

In other words, I'm a firm believer that most injuries can be avoided.

CHAPTER 19

THE CORE PROBLEM

The term *core* has been thrown around a great deal over the last few years, as in, "You have to get your core strong," or "Your back hurts because you have a weak core," or "Core training will help you play better tennis."

These statements and many others about core strength can be very misleading, and even potentially damaging due to a misunderstanding of the underlying issue creating pain or poor performance. A weak core should not be the default scapegoat for poor performance or injury.

Your core is defined by many health professionals as your abs, specifically your transverse abdominis, your obliques, your spinal erector muscles, and the muscles of your midsection. Some people include the glutes and hip flexors in their definition, but almost all agree that a strong core means a stable spine.

Many trainers preach that strengthening core muscles will make you will feel better, move better, produce more power, and generally be much better off. Unfortunately, that's not always true.

What all those things really require is a *balanced* core. In laymens' terms, that means the muscles surrounding the shoulders, rib cage, and hips should all be under equal and balanced tension like the strings on a marionet puppet that are pulled taut on all sides.

Let me explain the difference between balanced versus strong. When you have an elevated and rotated pelvis (*Fig. 19.1 below*), as many people do, you have an imbalance of tension and pressure on both hips and your low back. In fact, your back is more compressed on the elevated side. That compression leads to pressure on the lumbar discs, which consequently displace and herniate (slip). A strong core doesn't change the imbalance, because no matter how strong you are, the hip is still elevated and there's still pressure on the discs to slip.

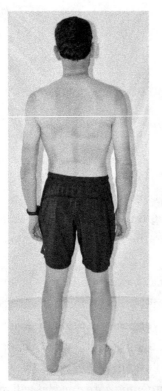

Figure 19.1 Notice the elevated hip on the left side. That's not just his shorts; on palpation of his pelvis, it truly is higher than on his right side. This is a world champion athlete, and despite having what most would consider a strong core, he still can't run without triggering back pain. Yet.

Here's another example of why *strong* doesn't signify *stable* (and there are a hundred to choose from). It's very common for the dominant shoulder of tennis players to drop forward and down (*Fig. 19.2*). When that shoulder drops it creates tension on one side of the neck and compression on one side of the lower back, creating imbalanced pressure on those vertebral discs, which again leaves them vulnerable to slip out of place. The shoulder drop also leaves imbalanced tension on each side of the spine, which then causes the upper body and pelvis to rotate.

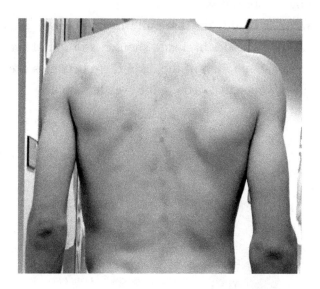

Figure 19.2 Notice how much lower the right shoulder is from the left, also evident from how much lower the right elbow sits compared to the opposite side. You can also see the right shoulder blade sitting lower and more defined, and more definition on the right side of the muscles of his back. This is typical in right-handed tennis players at all levels.

This in turn creates torque in your lower back, or upper back, or even in your knee. A strong core doesn't touch any of these imbalances, and attempting to strengthen anything without addressing the rotation or the position of the dropped shoulder and the corresponding shoulder blade is counterproductive at best.

One last example to drive the point home. When your upper back is rounded forward, or if your pelvis is tucked under out of its neutral position (*Fig. 19.3*), there is compression on your neck, stress on the lumbar spine, and the diaphragm's full ability to function is completely compromised.

Unfortunately, in these situations typical exercises focused on strengthening the core usually make all those things worse. The reason is most people focus on strengthening the abs rather than changing the position of the thoracic back, and they don't think of restoring the lumbar curve.

The result is tighter abs that pull the pelvis under even more, which triggers the upper back and shoulders to round even more forward, and the function of the diaphragm becomes even more compromised, which makes the spine even less stable.

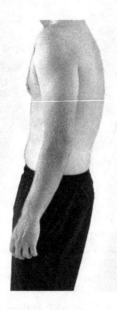

Figure 19.3 Showing both upper back rounding, and tucked under (posteriorly tilted) hips, which compromises breathing and the spine's ability to bear weight properly. You can't achieve true core strength until this posture is balanced out.

In all these situations, which are extremely common, just strengthening the muscles of the trunk and midsection usually make the imbalances worse while increasing the chance of injury.

I was a perfect example of someone who was strong but still unstable. When my back was constantly locking up in college, I went to doctors and trainers who practically unanimously recommended I strengthen my abs and stretch my hamstrings. Yet, I could do a thousand sit-ups and palm the ground without bending my knees, and I still hurt.

In fact, the more sit-ups I did, the more my back hurt. It turns out the sit-ups were only increasing an existing imbalance. I had an elevated right hip (Fig. *19.1)*, my abs and hip flexors were way too tight, and my mid back was rounded forward rather than lining up with my lower and upper back. The sit-ups were only making my hips tighter, and the strengthening exercises targeting my back only further fatigued my already overworked and stressed low back muscles.

Nobody warned me I might get tighter as I attempted to become stronger because they really didn't know what was causing my back pain.

This lack of understanding of cause and effect and the propensity to treat the symptom are exactly why the current Western medical model is so challenged and inefficient at treating chronic musculoskeletal pain. The result is millions of dollars and precious time wasted on MRIs, drugs, and unnecessary surgeries, and just as many frustrated patients that are still in pain and looking for answers.

You don't need an MRI to detect imbalance. The position of your shoulders, hips, knees, and ankles will tell you all you need to know. When they're stacked up and in their neutral positions, you'll be as strong as you need to be to play tennis and to live your life without pain or limitation.

The exercises in the *Totally Balanced Tennis Player Routine* and the functional strength routines that follow are purposely designed to help you accomplish those goals.

CHAPTER 20

THE TENNIS COMMANDMENTS

Most of us are guilty of some common stroke and movement faults from time to time. When I was growing up, my coaches yelled at me to stay down on my backhand, keep my racket on the ball, keep my head up on my serve, stay on balance, and other such tennis commandments.

Does any of this advice sound familiar? Have you ever wanted to wring your coach's neck after being yelled at again and again to "move your feet"? I often felt that way.

It turns out, the big reason I couldn't heed my coach's wise advice was my inability to transfer weight properly to my right hip. Most of you are unwittingly doing the same thing because I see it at all levels and at every club I've ever played in over the last twenty years, which is about how long I've been tracking it.

My imbalance stemmed from an injury I incurred over the summer after third grade. I was playing tackle football with some of the kids from our neighborhood outside Denver, where I grew up. I intercepted a ball and began to run when two boys tackled me from the side. The next thing I remember is getting loaded into an ambulance with a broken right leg. At nine years old I had managed to fracture my femur, the biggest bone in the body.

My older sister, who threw the pass I intercepted, said she heard the crack when my leg broke from about twenty yards away. The impressive injury earned me three weeks of healing in the hospital followed by four weeks in a full-body cast up to my chest. That's seven weeks of zero muscle activity on that leg.

When the cast was finally removed my right leg was half the size and half the strength of my left leg. As I slowly returned to tennis my brain subconsciously wouldn't let me transfer all my weight to my right leg because it detected the weakness.

Unfortunately, I quickly learned to work around that weakness by forming habits that became very hard to break. For example, I learned to turn out of my forehand prematurely to get me off my right leg as soon as possible. I noticed it especially when I got nervous during a match.

Over time, my body adapted to this habit by rotating my right hip forward even when I wasn't playing tennis. My right knee then followed by turning inward because the hip and knee share the same bone, the femur. As a result of both my right hip and my right knee falling out of their neutral positions, my right shoulder dropped forward and down because it lost its base of support. (See *Figs. 19.1* and *19.2* in the previous chapter.)

The next thing I knew, I had tons of trouble keeping my head up on my serve because my dropped shoulder wanted to pull me forward and down instead of staying up.

If this sounds complicated, it's really not. As I keep saying, nothing happens in isolation when it comes to the positional change of a major load joint like the shoulder, knee, hip, or ankle.

So now that you've done the self-assessment, how do you think your body compensates on the tennis court as a result of your imbalances?

You don't have to have all the answers, but do take time to think about it. I gave you an example earlier in the book about the junior player who lacked power on his serve due to his right knee collapsing in during his knee bend. His knee was compensating for a weak right hip.

You have your own compensations that are impeding your ability to get the most out of your game and are creating some common flaws in your mechanics. Examples include dropping your head on your serve, not bending your knees enough, and others. When that happens, your pro offers up some tips to fix them. I call these tips *commandments* because they're so common and all-encompassing, and if you violate them you're in danger of joining those other poor souls in tennis-loser purgatory. Unfortunately, as good as your pro's advice may be, sometimes there is no lasting solution until you fix your body first.

Here are some common commandments that I hear from pros all the time, the musculoskeletal culprits driving them, and some quick-fix solutions:

Reach up more on your serve

Failure to reach up fully on your serve or coming over the top of it rather than hitting "up" usually means you have a shoulder blade that isn't rotating fully, and a shoulder joint that isn't reaching its full range of motion. It also means that same side hip joint is a little stuck, and/ or your upper back is too rounded. This routine will address all those issues and will take you three minutes.

KNEELING GROIN STRETCH
Duration: 1 minute each side

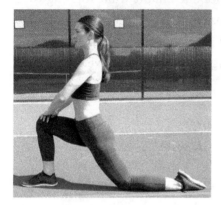

Begin by kneeling on the ground on both knees; then step forward into a lunge position. Keep your upper body straight and sink your hips down toward the ground until you feel a stretch on the front of your trailing leg. Relax your shoulders and your stomach.

KNEELING WALL CLOCK
Duration: 1 minute each position

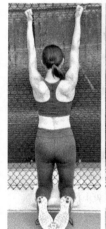 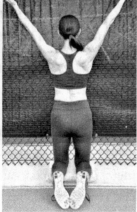 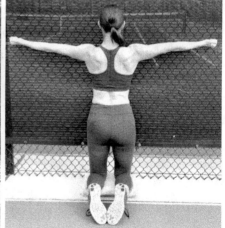

Position 1   *Position 2*   *Position 3*

As you can see there are three positions. Start with your knees and forehead touching the wall or fence and bring your arms straight up above you. Make a light fist with your thumbs pointed out and rotate your arms out from the shoulder. Make sure you drop your shoulders down away from your ears, keep your elbows locked, and pigeon-toe your feet. Relax your stomach. After a minute bring your arms out to 45 degrees and hold for one minute while rotating your thumbs out. Then bring your arms straight out from your shoulders for the final minute. This exercise engages all the stabilizing muscles of your shoulders while realigning your upper back over your hips.

Stay down on everything: forehand, backhand, volleys

The real issue is that you're pulling up early, which means you're not transferring your weight properly to your front foot.

These exercises done together should take you a total of five minutes. They retrain your nervous system to balance out the weight distribution in your hips.

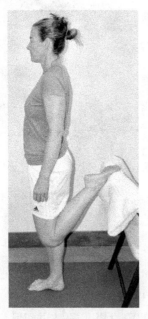

STANDING QUAD STRETCH
Duration: 1 minute each leg

Put your leg up behind you on a chair, couch, or the net if you're on the court. Keep your upper body straight, your bent knee right next to the straight leg (don't let your bent knee flare out to the side). Tuck your hips under to increase the stretch on your thigh. This exercise reminds each hip of its ability to bear weight while asking the upper body to stay out of the way.

KNEELING GROIN STRETCH WITH OVERHEAD EXTENSION
Duration: 1 minute each side

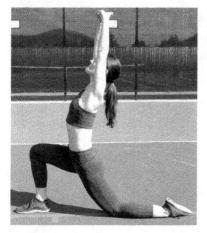

Go into a lunge position with the knee of your back leg on the ground. Sink your hips down toward the ground until you feel a stretch on the front of your trailing hip. Interlace your fingers together with palms away from you and pull your hands up and above your head with your arms straight. Hold the position. This exercise reminds each hip to balance and bear load while making sure the upper back can't help.

FREE SQUAT
Duration 30 seconds to 1 minute

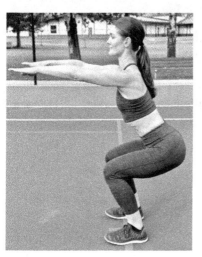

With both feet straight and hip-width apart squat down by dropping your hips to just above 90 degrees. Keep an arch in your low back, look straight ahead and keep your upper body up (try not to lean forward). This exercise resets the trunk over the hips and forces the body to evenly weight both sides. It also gives you practice on staying down!

Turn your shoulders more

Rotating your trunk, or lack thereof, is indicative of the function and position of your lower and mid back, as well as the mobility of your hips. Not turning enough means you're trying to do everything with your arm rather than incorporating the entire chain of muscles from your hips to your fingers. Tennis is a sport driven from the hips, and shoulder turn is always initiated by the hips and shoulders rotating together.

This sequence should also take you about five minutes total, and it will prepare your back for rotation and shoulder turn.

STATIC EXTENSION POSITION
Duration: 1 to 2 Minutes

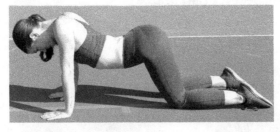

While on your hands and knees, walk your hands forward until your hips are four to six inches in front of your knees. Keep your hands directly under your shoulders and let your shoulder blades drop together while you allow your chest to drop toward the ground. Keep your elbows straight and relax your chin down toward your chest. DO NOT MOVE YOUR HIPS TOO FAR FORWARD. If you feel you're in a modified push-up or your hips have dropped below your shoulders, you've probably gone too far.

Upper Spinal Floor Twist
Duration: 1 minute per side

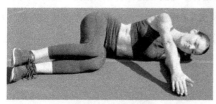

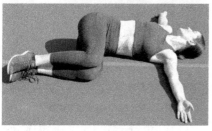

Lie on one side with your knees and hips at 90 degrees and your knees and ankles stacked together. Without letting your knees come apart or slide off one another, open your top arm up to the opposite side keeping your palm up. Look toward your open hand and breathe! As you exhale let your arm and the back of your hand drop toward the ground. Your head should be comfortably on the ground. If not, place a pillow under your head. This exercise reminds your spine of its ability to rotate while opening up your mid and upper back.

Overhead Extension Feet Pigeon-Toed
Duration: 1 minute

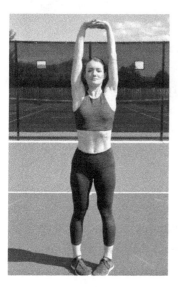

Stand with your feet pigeon-toed, stomach relaxed. Keep the weight on the insides of your feet and tighten your thighs. Interlace your hands together with palms facing out and pull your arms up straight overhead like you're reaching for the sky. Keep your hips over your ankles instead of letting them thrust forward. This exercise restores the link between your lower body and upper body. It also repositions all your major load joints under vertical load again.

Bend your knees

This is different from staying down because it implies that you never got down to begin with. Not bending your knees is a sign of hips delegating their responsibility of stability and function to the upper body.

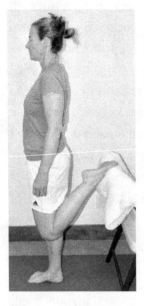

STANDING QUAD STRETCH
Duration: 1 minute each side

With one foot behind you on a chair, a couch, or the net if you're on the court, tuck your hips under until you feel a stretch on the front of your thigh. Keep your bent knee next to, and in line with, the other. When you look down at your knees, they should be even rather than one in front of the other. Keep your upper body straight and the foot on your standing leg pointing straight ahead. The purpose of this is to restore hip function and stability.

STATIC EXTENSION POSITION

See page 211 for instructions. The purpose here is to restore the natural bend and curve to your spine, which allows you to keep your upper body upright as your knees flex.

Keep your head up

Your head is attached to your neck and your neck is attached to your upper back. Therefore, pulling your head down is a symptom of forward rounded shoulders and/or a rounded upper back.

This sequence will take you about three minutes and will free up your upper back so you can keep your head up when serving or hitting an overhead.

KNEELING MODIFIED COUNTER STRETCH
Duration: 1 minute

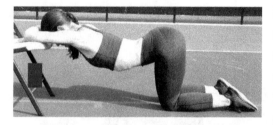

Kneel in front of a chair or couch. Rest your arms with elbows bent and arms crossed on the edge of a chair or couch. Rest your head on the chair, walk your knees back until they're directly under your hips and let your back sway like you're allowing an arch to form. Relax your stomach, let your chest and stomach relax toward the ground. This exercise opens up your chest and realigns your upper back while reconnecting the extensor muscles on your spine from top to bottom.

CROCODILE
Duration: 1 minute each side

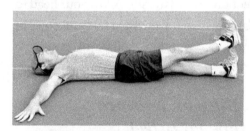

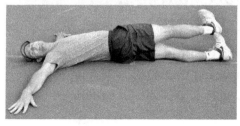

With both legs straight rest the heel of one foot on top of the toes of the other. Your arms should be straight out from your shoulders, palms down. Keeping your thighs tight, knees locked and feet flexed back toward you, roll your hips over in the direction of your bottom leg. Look the opposite way and hold. Roll as much as you can, keeping both shoulders on the ground and your knees locked. Don't shift your hips to make the roll easier. This should feel like work as you're reconnecting the whole backside of your body while asking your lower and upper back to extend and rotate just like they would while hitting a serve.

CATS AND DOGS
Reps: 10

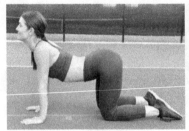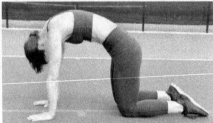

On all fours with your hands directly under your shoulders and knees directly under your hips, let your back sway and your shoulder blades glide together as your chest and stomach drop toward the ground. Keep your elbows locked out. Let your head come up as your stomach and back drop down. Don't hold as you change directions, rounding your back in the opposite direction toward the sky. Allow your head to drop as your back rounds. Cats and dogs, also called "cat and cow" in yoga, restores symmetrical motion to your hips, spine and shoulders.

Keep your balance. Stay on balance through the shot. Move your feet.

Multiple commandments here with the same cause. Falling off balance and not moving your feet are signs of improper weight transfer, unstable or tight hips, and that you're reaching with your arm rather than moving your feet to the ball. This routine will take you three minutes.

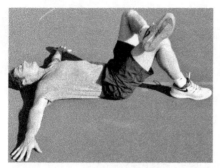

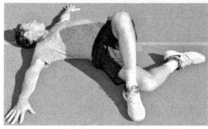

Hip Crossover Stretch
Duration: 1 minute each side

Lie on your back with your knees bent and arms straight out from your shoulders. Keep your palms down. Cross one ankle over the other knee, and then drop that foot and the outside of the bottom leg to the ground. Keep that ankle glued to the opposite knee and don't shift the foot on the ground—just roll. Once in position, use your leg muscles to push the knee sticking up in the air away from you. You should feel a stretch in the outside of your hip or thigh. This exercise prepares your hips to move from side to side.

Core Abs 1st Position
Duration: 30 seconds to 1 minute

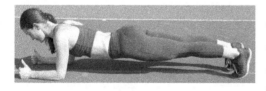

This position is like a traditional plank on your elbows with two big exceptions: Your hands are shoulder-width apart with your thumbs up, and your shoulder blades are squeezed together. Squeezed HARD! Your hips will want to drop toward the ground, but don't let them. It's imperative you keep your hips level with your shoulders and your legs locked with thighs contracted. This exercise is balancing out the muscles on the front side of your body with those on the backside and asking for major stability and strength from your hips. If there's too much stress in your low back, tighten up your stomach muscles and flatten your low back a bit to decrease some of the arch.

These are the major common coaching tips I hear from the pros, but of course, there are plenty more. If I didn't mention your challenge, then pick one of the above that it most closely resembles. As I mentioned before, any positive positional change to any major joint will affect all the major load joints, so these exercises will likely address any challenge you'd like to tackle.

PART IV

SOLUTIONS FOR COMMON AILMENTS

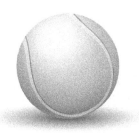

CHAPTER 21

THE FOUR HORSEMAN OF BACK PAIN

Because of my struggle with back pain when I was in high school and college, I truly empathize with those of you who are also engaged in your own frustrating battle with back issues. An aching back is not fun, and it's not conducive to playing your best tennis; nor is any pain or injury for that matter.

There are four major postural causes that lead to mechanical dysfunctions of low-back pain. These same alignment issues can also lead to mid- or upper-back pain. I've included the undesirable tennis consequences that go along with these postures to highlight how much your game will improve once you fix your alignment with the exercises.

Tennis demands a lot from our backs. We bend forward while reaching for low balls, we twist to hit every stroke, we bend backward to serve or to hit an overhead, and we laterally flex our spines for just about every stroke. In other words, our backs are constantly engaged in some degree of flexion, extension or rotation while playing. Keep in mind, though, that we're designed to do it. Therefore, in order to be pain-free and to tap into your dazzling athleticism, it's imperative that your hips and spine stay pliable and completely functional while also stacking up with your other load-bearing joints.

A quick discussion on spinal anatomy: We are a unique species in that not only are we bipedal, but our pelvis is more bowl shaped compared to any other animal. It's shaped that way in order accommodate a vertical rather than horizontal spine, and to carry all the weight of the upper body and displace it over two limbs rather than over four.

Like a Roman or Greek column, the vertical alignment of our spines allows for stability and even transfer of force from top to bottom. Unlike a marble or stone column, though, our spine also moves.

For this reason, our spines are segmented via vertebrae, and together as a unit they form the shape of an *S*. The shape acts as a spring that absorbs force and limits compression (Fig. *21.1*). If you push down on a spring, it will compress. If you push down at an angle, the spring will compress and bulge on one side to accommodate and absorb the pressure. Our spines do the same thing, which is why spinal pliability is imperative. The pliability comes from the somewhat elastic property of muscles, tendons and ligaments, but also from the space between the vertebrae.

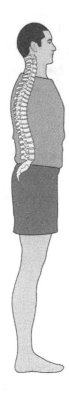

Figure 21.1 The S curve of the spine allowing for both motion and stability.

In summation, when it comes to a healthy back, think vertical alignment with S-curve and flexibility.

With that in mind, here are the four common postural causes of back pain:

The First Horseman: Losing the S Curve

Each individual vertebra allows for 2 degrees of rotation and is set far enough apart to bend, twist, and turn without bumping up against the bone above or below it. Up to a point of course.

However, that end point is dramatically reduced if the discs between the vertebrae have shrunk (due to dehydration or poor spinal alignment), or if the *S* curve has been modified or changed in any way.

Have you ever heard the term, "Flat back with a crack?" It's used to describe someone who doesn't appear to have much of a butt (*Fig. 21.2*). But it's really describing someone whose hips have tucked under and who has lost the normal and necessary curve in their lower back.

Once the spine flattens out, the intervertebral discs begin to be squashed rather than merely compressed, which greatly increases their rate of deterioration. Degenerative discs are the result, which further impedes shock absorption and movement because the more the discs wear out and compress, the less space the vertebrae have to move. Pain usually follows either from back muscles that are fatigued from being elongated all day long, and/or from being compressed and irritated spinal soft tissue.

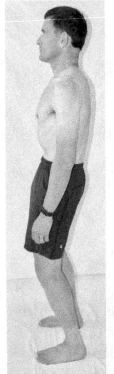

Notice the lack of curve in the lower back where the spine becomes more of a rigid column than a shock-absorbing spring. (*Fig. 21.2*)

As a tennis player, losing your spinal curve (and your booty shelf) is a problem. Bending, twisting, turning, reaching, footwork, and moving in general will suffer. In a nutshell, you'll lose 90 percent or more of your athleticism. The solution is to restore the *S* curve with exercises that trigger the back muscles and hip muscles to rebalance with each other, and to reposition the shoulders so they align directly over the hips. The final phase will be to restore motion to a body that's been starving for it.

Figure 21.2

The Second Horseman: Rounded Shoulders and/or a Rounded Upper Back

If you have a rounded upper back or forward rounding shoulders, lower back pain won't be far behind (plus likely neck pain). Even if you have a perfect curve in your lower back, if the upper back rounds forward, the lower back muscles automatically have to grab on to provide a counterbalance so you don't fall over.

Those back muscles don't appreciate the extra stress and work for long periods of time any more than you would appreciate holding a ten-pound weight in your hand all day long. As the back muscles fatigue, they begin to burn and hurt, which is exactly what tired muscles do when they're screaming for a break.

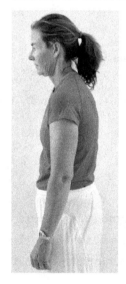

Unfortunately, the most common treatment for back pain is to strengthen back muscles and abs. I guess if they get stronger, they might be able to hold out longer, but they're more likely to just get tighter and even more fatigued. Either way, it's still a losing battle until the upper back gets out of flexion (stops rounding). So, why not address the real problem to begin with?

The consequences to your tennis game of a rounded upper back or of slouching shoulders are many: Decreased range of motion and function of your entire spine, shoulder joints, elbows and wrists, diminished power on your serve and groundstrokes due to a more restricted swing motion, a propensity to pull your head down on your serve, and dipping your upper body forward to reach for low balls, as opposed to bending your knees, are all likely results.

The Third Horseman: Rotated Hips/Elevated Hip

Another contributor to back pain is a pelvis that's rotated or elevated on one side (*Fig. 21.4*). This should sound familiar to many of you, especially if anyone has ever mentioned they have "one leg longer than the other." In my experience that's often not the case. Legs are the same length 99 percent of the time. The discrepancy is actually due to a muscle imbalance causing a pelvic rotation. The result is one leg bone is sitting in a different place in the hip joint compared to the other leg, which makes it appear longer.

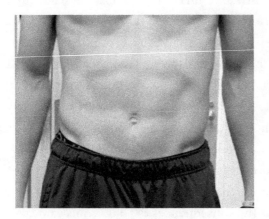

Figure 21.4 Observe the right hip. You can clearly see the elevation and rotation on that side.

The practitioner who told you one leg is longer often knows better and adjusts you to even things out. However, the adjustment rarely holds because you have a muscle memory and other imbalances that pull your hips back out of alignment.

Considering birth defects affecting leg length are extremely rare, the only reasons you would have one leg actually longer is if you broke your leg during your growing years, which can disrupt the growth plate, or if you were the unfortunate recipient of a broken pelvis. In these cases, where there is a marked discrepancy between actual bone length, a lift in your shoe might be warranted.

An elevated or rotated hip creates compression on one side of the spine. Remember, the spine is designed to sit over a level pelvis, and the muscles around the spine are supposed to create equal tension on the spine. As soon as you elevate or rotate one side, you disrupt the spinal muscle tension and increase the spinal pressure on one side. The result is often a bulging disc (or multiple bulging discs).

Unfortunately, shoulders that aren't level can have the same effect as uneven hips because they also increase the spinal tension and compression on one side. Again, the treatment shouldn't focus on strengthening the back muscles. In fact, the more you strengthen the muscles with a pelvis that's not level, the more you run the risk of reinforcing the imbalance.

First, you must get the hips and shoulders more level by taking the rotation out of the pelvis, and by balancing the muscles in and around the hips. Once you have symmetry and balance you can strengthen your back all you want—although you probably won't have to.

The tennis consequences of an imbalanced pelvic girdle are numerous. One common symptom is a slower reaction time when moving to one side while returning serve, or while moving to one side for a groundstroke. For instance, if your weight distribution is more on your right leg (rather than equally distributed between both) you'll move better to your left. You always move better toward your disfunction, which, in this case, is a weak left hip.

Try it yourself. Get into your return stance and put slightly more weight in your right leg. Now imagine someone has hit a serve to your left (toward your backhand if you're a righty) and spring over to get it. Notice the quick reaction. Now put more weight on your right again in your stance and try to spring to your right (your forehand for a righty) as you would to retrieve a slice serve in the deuce court. Pay attention again to your reaction time. You'll notice that in order to move, you had to first transfer your weight to your left leg so you could push off your left in order to move right, or you had to awkwardly cross over your other leg, which decreased your reach by a foot or more. Transferring enough weight to the opposite leg robs precious milliseconds that could mean getting to the ball slightly late, or not getting to it at all.

Players at all levels are affected by uneven weight distribution in the hips, and thus a slow reaction time while moving to one side. But the bigger your opponent's serve, the less time you have. Therefore, I can't overly state the importance of being evenly balanced while returning serve, when split-stepping on your way to the net, or while in your ready position during the point.

The Fourth Horseman: Sway Back

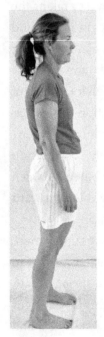

The final major postural contributor to back pain is poor alignment of the hips in relation to the shoulders and ankles. We call this *forward sway*, or sometimes called *sway back* (*Fig. 21.5*). It means that if you were looking at yourself from the side view, your hips would appear to be forward of your shoulders and ankles. The problem with sway-back posture is that instead of the force of gravity going through your spine equally from top to bottom, it displaces the stress all on your lower back. The alignment is akin to doing a backbend all day long. No wonder your muscles ache!

The other problem with sway back is that it means your center of gravity, which lies just above your hip joint, has shifted forward. That shift causes your upper back or shoulders to round forward and

Figure 21.5

your head to move forward to rebalance itself. That's why forward hips and neck pain/shoulder pain almost always go hand in hand.

Unfortunately, too many people think their neck pain is a separate and independent issue from their back pain. It's not, and never is. The neck and shoulders are connected to the same spine as the hips and lower back. If there's a problem with one, there's a problem with the other, even if the discomfort is only in one and not the other.

The cure is to trigger the deep hip stabilizers to re-center your hips under your shoulders and over your ankles.

The exercises I give you will do exactly that without you having to consciously think about holding your hips back over your ankles all day.

Forward sway has many tennis consequences, led by a very slow response to moving forward. Reacting to short balls is particularly affected because without the hips being underneath you, your center of gravity has to come back before you can move forward. With every unnecessary movement you're losing precious time.

General instability and lack of power are also common with this posture because the weak hip muscles can't offer a strong base of support.

If you have any form of back pain, follow these exercises daily in the order they appear. They're designed to address all the major postural imbalances contributing to, or likely causing, your back pain. They'll also get you moving better and feeling better on the tennis court. Once the pain abates, you can continue with this menu as your daily routine, or you can move on to the overall *Totally Balanced Tennis Player* daily or strength menus that come later in this book.

This sequence should take you fifteen to twenty minutes total. Do it every day if you're in pain.

KNEELING MODIFIED COUNTER STRETCH
Duration: 1 minute

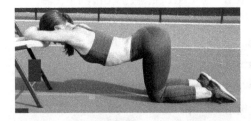

Kneel and rest your elbows and forearms on a chair or couch with elbows bent and arms crossed. Bring your knees directly under your hips. Let your back sway as you allow your chest and stomach to drop toward the ground. This exercise repositions your mid and upper back and reconnects all the extensors of your spine.

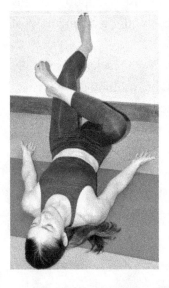

ASSISTED HIP LIFT
Duration: 1 minute per side

This exercise reduces the rotation in your hips. Lie on your back with your feet on the wall and knees bent 90 degrees. Cross one ankle over the other knee and use your leg muscles (not your hand) to press your knee away from you toward the wall. Keep the foot on the wall straight, both hips evenly on the ground, and make sure your hips stay level as you cross your ankle over and especially as you push your knee away. You'll feel this in your glute and the outside of your leg. Relax your arms and shoulders with your palms up out to the sides.

Static Back
Duration: 5 to 10 minutes

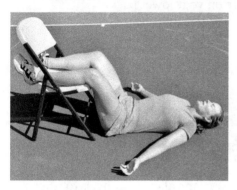

This wonderfully relaxing position allows the muscles of your hips and spine to take a break and to balance out the tension from top to bottom and front to back. The key is to put your legs up as close to 90 degrees at the knees and hips as possible. Relax your shoulders, put your palms up and out to the sides. Make sure your arms are resting below your shoulders but not too low. Breathe by allowing your stomach to rise as you inhale and let your stomach fall as you exhale. Notice the pressure of your back on the ground. It should feel evenly weighted from the low back to the upper back. If not, that's okay; it will eventually settle.

Static Back Pullovers
Reps: 30

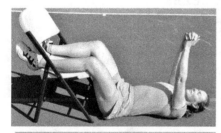

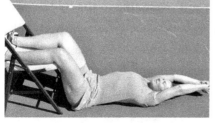

While in the static back position, place your palms together and interlace your fingers. Keeping your elbows straight, pull your arms up overhead as far as they go without bending the elbows. Try to hit the ground above your head if you can, without bending your elbows. Bring your arms up and back thirty times and notice it gets easier as you go. The pullovers restore function to the shoulders while helping to balance out the spinal muscles. They also help realign your upper back to take the pressure off your lower back.

Cobra on Elbows
Duration: 1 minute

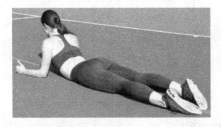

Lie on your stomach with your elbows directly underneath your shoulders. Pigeon toe your feet and allow your heels to relax out away from each other. Make a fist with your thumbs up and pry your hands away from one another. Allow your chest to drop toward the ground and slide your shoulder blades together. Hold. This exercise reminds your spine of its ability to find uniform extension (bending back) rather than doing so in pieces and parts. Make sure your shoulder blades squeeze down and back away from your ears.

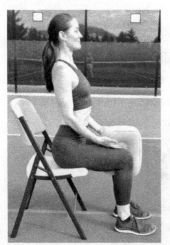

Sitting Knee Pillow Squeezes
Reps: 60

This exercise will tire out your inner thighs while strengthening the stabilizing muscles of your hips, which play an integral role in supporting your back. Start by sitting in the middle of a chair or bench, align your ankles directly under your knees to form a right angle at your knees and hips. Keep your feet straight and roll your hips forward to create an arch in your low back.

Don't just arch your back. Use the muscles on the front of your hips (your hip flexors) to roll the hips forward. Keep your upper body straight and directly over your hips. Relax your shoulders and squeeze the pillow with even pressure. You can use a pillow from your bed or couch, a yoga block, or anything that keeps your knees about one to two fists-width apart.

AIRBENCH
Duration 1 to 2 minutes

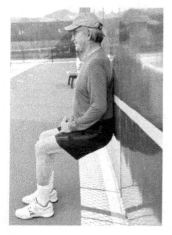

It's okay if you don't get to two minutes on your first try. I've worked with many pro athletes who practically shed tears after one minute. You'll get stronger quickly, though, and should be able to hold it for two minutes easily within a few weeks. The key is to drop to just above 90 degrees, press your low back firmly into the wall to eliminate any space between your back and the wall, keep your feet straight and about one to two fist-widths apart. Make sure your knees sit over your ankles rather than your toes. Keep the weight in your heels and use your legs to press your back into the wall. Enjoy.

Medical Symptoms of Misalignment

There are many other physical symptoms of a spine that's not neutrally aligned or not functioning as a unit. The allopathic world, also known as the Western medical model of health, usually treats these symptoms as causes, often mislabeling them as diseases. Yet, they are symptoms of misaligned shoulders and hips, which create havoc in the spine. Examples of medical diagnoses include stenosis, degenerative disc disease, disc bulges and disc herniations, sciatic pain, and spondylolisthesis.

Each one of these conditions commonly stems from an overload of compression on one side, or on one area of the spine—all due to your alignment. By fixing the underlying compression, or more accurately, the postural imbalance causing the compression, you can vastly improve or often fix the condition. In other words, treat the position of your body rather than the condition (the symptom), and the pain usually disappears.

I'm not saying other treatments won't be helpful or sometimes needed, but I am saying you might want to address a major contributing factor if not the cause—your posture—along the way.

CHAPTER 22

THE TWIST IN YOUR SHOULDER, ELBOW, AND WRIST

I've combined shoulder, elbow and wrist pain in the same chapter because they function as one unit. You can't rotate your upper arm bone without affecting your elbow and wrist any more than you can rotate your hip joint without moving your knee and ankle. The wrist bones are connected to the elbow bones, which are connected to the shoulder bones. These parts function together, so they should also be treated together.

Today's modern forehand is a perfect example of the intertwined relationship of the entire muscular chain from the shoulder blade all the way to the wrist. Rather than the low-to-high idea of brushing up on the ball to create topspin, the new rackets, Western grips, and synthetic strings have ushered in a new era of stroke mechanics.

The forehand is now about tremendous external rotation of the arm followed by massive internal rotation of the shoulder, elbow and wrist. The elbow now routinely ends up being above the wrist at the finish, which was almost impossible with the wood rackets and the strokes of the champions of old. The result is heavy spin, devastating power, and massive torque on the entire arm. I know what you're thinking: *"No wonder there's so much pain!"* I agree, but it's not because of the stroke, it's because of the body going into the stroke. We're designed to do it; otherwise, we wouldn't.

A functional shoulder can handle the extra stress and demand, but a dysfunctional one will pass the buck along to the elbow or the wrist (or both) to compensate. For example, if the shoulder joint doesn't rotate completely to allow the upper arm bone to go from external rotation to its full range of internal rotation and pronation of the hand, the bones of the forearm will have to rotate excessively instead.

Excessive forearm rotation creates strain on the muscles and tendons of the elbow. If the elbow isn't up to the task, then the wrist bears the brunt of rotation, putting stress on those tendons and ligaments.

By the way, the old strokes produced their share of arm and elbow pain as well, and people blamed the heavy rackets back then. As a result, new technology surfaces every year now to minimize or deaden the impact that passes from your racket to your wrist and forearm. However, neither softer strings, sand in the racket head, a lighter racket, a shock absorber, carbon fiber technology, or any other technological breakthrough can compensate for a lack of shoulder function.

I'm not saying all that new technology can't help; I'm sure there are numerous studies and tons of data proving it can. However, all the technology in the world doesn't come close to beating the brilliant design of the human body, and we still have to treat the cause of the pain, not just mitigate the symptom.

To illustrate how much stronger the muscles and bones are when working together rather than individually, let's do a quick test; you're going to squeeze someone's hand, or your own hand if needed. If you have a partner, round your shoulder noticeably forward, go to shake hands and squeeze. Exaggerate the forward rounding a little.

If it's your own hand you're squeezing and you're a righty, wrap your fingers around your left hand, let your right shoulder round forward, and squeeze as hard as you can.

Let your fingers in the hand being squeezed relax (don't hurt yourself). Notice the amount of force and strength you can produce. Now pull your right shoulder blade back, which pulls your right shoulder in line. Now squeeze as hard as you can. You should notice that with your shoulder pulled back you can produce much more force. You'll probably notice that you recruit more or different muscles to do the squeezing.

You're stronger with your shoulder pulled back because now your entire arm can get in on the action. The shoulder, elbow, wrist and hand are now all working together as a unit to accomplish the task rather than just the hand muscles or the muscles of the forearm.

Now imagine gripping a racket and hitting a tennis ball with this same feeling of the entire muscular chain (your hand to your shoulder and beyond) working together as a unit. You would exert much less effort while producing much more power on each and every stroke.

The exercises here are designed to treat the wrist, elbow and shoulder as a unit, but how we treat it can vary depending on what we can get away with based on the actual symptom. In other words, if you have a torn rotator cuff, you might not be able to do the same exercises you can do if you have wrist pain.

Therefore, I've broken up the menus into categories based on common tennis injuries and symptoms. You'll notice there are separate menus here for tennis elbow, shoulder pain, and wrist pain.

Of course, *always* pay attention to your instincts. When the pain is gone, go to the overall functional tennis player routine and/or to the strength routines as your daily menus. You can always come back to these specific pain menus anytime.

Tennis Elbow

Tennis elbow has become so common among recreational players that most people expect to get it at some time in their career. It doesn't have to be that way though. Technically, tennis elbow is an inflammation of the tendons and muscles of the forearm that attach to the outer elbow bone (lateral condyle). We'll just call it outer elbow and forearm pain for now. It's very fixable, but you must fix the *why* of the pain, which always ties in to the shoulder.

Let's go over some quick anatomy first to better understand how the elbow and shoulder bones function together.

The lower bones of the forearm (the ulna and radius) always rotate together and are designed to allow for rotation of the wrist, and pronation and supination of your hand (rolling your palm up or down).

To illustrate their connection to the shoulder, put your hands straight out in front of you (don't rest them on the table) and rotate your palms up toward the sky, then rotate them down toward the floor. Notice that your entire arm has to move in order to rotate your palms up and down, and the movement comes mostly from the shoulder. Now take your shoulder out of play by bending your elbows.

Rotate your palms up and down and notice while there is still some rotation in your upper arm, it's much less and the muscles of your forearm work much harder to get the job done. This is an example of the elbow and wrist muscles and bones compensating for a lack of rotation of the shoulder joint.

In a serve or forehand, when the shoulder muscles are imbalanced or the joint is out of position, the forearm muscles have to work harder than normal because they aren't able to get help from their bigger and more powerful friends. If your friends abandoned you in a time of need, you'd get angry. Same with those muscles and tendons that surround your elbow. The pain you feel in your elbow and forearm is their expression of anger from being left alone, along with a plea to get some help from their shoulder muscle friends to come to the rescue.

The exercises for tennis elbow are designed to restore the rotational connection between the wrist, elbow, and shoulder, reminding them that they're designed to work together. These exercises will also make sure the shoulder and the upper back are in their neutral positions and sitting over stable hips. Without the hips as a stable base, the shoulders (and thus the elbow and wrist) have no chance. Therefore, when you see an exercise that appears to be for the hips, don't despair; I promise there's a purpose.

Do these exercises exactly in the order they appear.

STANDING UNILATERAL CHEST OPENERS
Reps and sets: 20 reps of 3 sets per arm

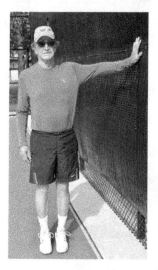

What you can't see in the picture is that he's rotating his elbow in and out while keeping his hand still. Start by standing sideways to a wall. Place your hand directly out from your shoulder to the side with your palm on the wall. Your fingers should be pointing toward the sky. Keep your elbow straight, your feet straight and relax your shoulders and neck. Rotate your elbow as far in and out as you can while keeping your shoulder down. Do twenty rotations, then switch arms. Repeat three times. This important exercise restores independent motion and rotation to your arm bones while reconnecting the muscles and bones from your hand to your shoulder. You might feel a slight stretch in your forearm, your chest muscles, or your upper arm.

CROCODILE
Duration: 1 minute each side

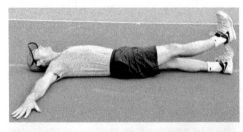
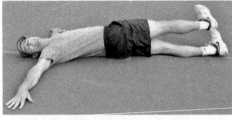

This is a great exercise to restore motion to your spine and to engage the stabilizing muscles in your shoulders and upper back. You might feel a stretch across your upper arm as you roll to the opposite side. Keep your thighs tight and knees locked out, feet pulled back, and arms straight out from your shoulders with your palms down. Place one heel on the other toe and roll toward the side with the down leg. Look the other way and keep both shoulders on the ground.

CATS AND DOGS
Reps: 10 cats and 10 dogs

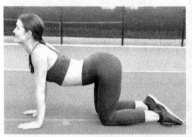
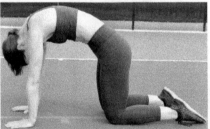

See page 66 for the instructions. These are reconnecting your hips and spine while also restoring motion to both. Remember to initiate the movement from your hips not your back.

WALL CLOCK
Duration: 1 minute each position

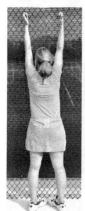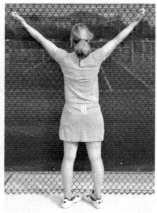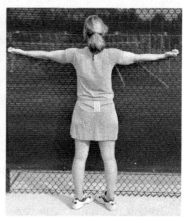

This is a phenomenal exercise to reconnect all the joints in your arm while strengthening the stabilizing muscles of your shoulders and upper back. Stand facing the wall with your feet pigeon-toed and toes touching the wall. Bring your arms straight up overhead for the first position, lock out your elbows, make a fist with your thumbs up and rotate your thumbs away from the wall by rotating from the shoulders. Hold 1 minute, then bring your arms to 45 degrees for one minute, then 90 degrees for the same time. Remember to keep your elbows straight, relax your shoulders down and back away from your neck, relax your stomach and feel the burn in those arms as they get stronger.

Shoulder pain

I treated my own shoulder for a rotator cuff tear in 2015. I was training for the National 40s Hardcourt Championships in La Jolla, and I failed to listen to my body. In preparation for the tournament, I went from training one to two days a week to four or five, and I hit buckets of serves to improve my accuracy. However, it's what I did off the court that caused the problem.

Tennis is an imbalanced sport, so the increased time and demand on the court meant I was becoming slightly more imbalanced. My right shoulder was doing more and more work and falling ever so slightly out of position. This might not have been a problem if I wasn't also swimming two days a week and doing some other functional strengthening in the gym.

Oh, I should also mention that I hadn't played a singles tournament in about five years.

The result was shoulder overload. The good news was I was feeling and playing great and I got to the semifinals. The bad news was by the time I reached the semis, my shoulder felt like a frayed piece of string that would unravel and break at the slightest hint of a mishit forehand or serve.

I had noticed my shoulder was feeling off and tired about ten days before the tournament, but I didn't think anything of it (I didn't listen to the whisper) because I figured that it wasn't serious. And with my knowledge and experience, I would fix it. I helped people solve pains like this every day, so wouldn't I surely solve my own? By the time I reached the quarterfinals my shoulder was so sore I could barely lift it, and after the match I knew it was time to take a break.

So, what did I do? I iced it, did some exercises, took some Advil, muted the pain, ignored my screaming shoulder, and played the semis.

There are three reasons I played on:

First, we're taught as young athletes to tough it out through the pain and ignore our body's messages, and I didn't want to feel like I was being weak or scared by backing out (ego).

Second, I figured I would fix anything that came up eventually because, after all, hasn't every injury I've ever had always healed (ego)?

Finally, I was really excited to play the semis and thought I could still potentially win, even with a compromised shoulder (ego).

Recognize a theme here?

At 2-2 in the first set I went to hit a first serve and the ball hit the baseline on the fly. I didn't feel pain, I just missed. Badly.

Then I did the same thing on the next point when my first serve almost hit my opponent on the fly. I realize now the fine motor control of my shoulder had abandoned me along with any ability to direct my first serve. I also noticed that I wasn't getting any power on my backhand (I'm a one-hander).

Perplexed but determined, I continued to play on, and lost convincingly. After the match I noticed that I couldn't get my right shoulder blade to retract completely. That's when the potential severity of the injury hit me.

After a month of trying to knock the pain and injury out using strengthening and other exercises with no luck, my good friend, who's also a shoulder doc, convinced me to get an MRI. The torn rotator cuff was obvious, but my shoulder also looked like it was dislocated, which is exactly how it felt. I didn't believe surgery was the answer for me, though, and I took it upon myself to try to fix it.

The first thing I did was take a month off and ice my shoulder two times per day. To the extent it could, my shoulder needed time and space to rest and heal. With the exception of some whole-body exercises I'll show you in this book, for an entire month there was no tennis, no bands or weights, no push-ups or pull-ups, no sit-ups, no anything that placed demands on my shoulder, other than normal activities. And my shoulder turned the corner.

After a month of rest, I got into exercises similar to the ones I'm giving you here, and before long I was playing tennis again. Although I could serve without pain at about 75 percent effort, it took me about a year to confidently serve at full speed.

This is where the moral of the story lies, and the three biggest points I want to make:

1. Get your ego out of the way and listen to your body.
2. Sometimes you just need to rest and let your body heal.
3. You can have a torn rotator cuff and not have pain.

You can also have a herniated disc, a torn meniscus in your knee, and other symptoms and not have pain. That is, you can potentially keep playing without issue as long as you restore the function and the position of your body to allow it to function as a unit again. That's not to say you should avoid surgery; that's up to you based on your instincts, how you feel, and the professional advice you get if you choose to seek it.

There is a time and a place for surgery, for sure, but I didn't feel like it was the right choice for me at the time and I'm glad for it now.

Possibly the most important lesson of all is to drop all ego and don't play through the pain. It's not worth it. Ever!

Whether you have a rotator cuff tear, or general shoulder pain, this menu will reposition your shoulder back to neutral. The major causes of shoulder pain are not your serve or slice backhand. The cause is a shoulder that's out of position, and not working in conjunction with your shoulder blade to rotate properly. Remember to think *position*, not *condition*, which is exactly how we're going to treat it.

STATIC WALL—REVERSE PRESSES
Reps: 30

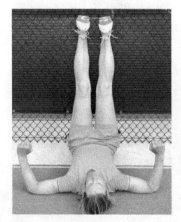

Lying on your back with your legs straight up a wall, place your elbows directly out from your shoulders with your elbows bent and fists in the air. Push your knees toward the wall, contract your thigh muscles and flex your feet and toes back toward your knees. Make sure the bottoms of your feet are flat instead of angled. You'll have to use the muscles on the outsides of your ankles to roll your feet straight. Imagine that you have a dinner plate filled with mashed potatoes resting on the bottoms of your feet. If you angle your feet, they'll slide right off that plate, but if you keep them perfectly flat, they'll hang out there. Once in position squeeze your shoulder blades together, then release them. Slide them together and down away from your ears. Repeat thirty times. This is an important exercise to restore the position and functional glide of your shoulder blades.

UPPER SPINAL FLOOR TWIST
Duration: 1 minute each side

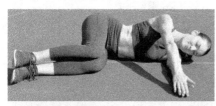
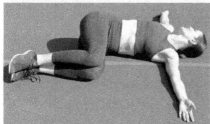

See instructions on page 92. This exercise is repositioning your upper back while also restoring proper glide to your shoulder blades. You might feel a stretch across your chest or even your low back. Breathe and let your open arm drop toward the ground as you exhale.

CATS AND DOGS

See pictures and instructions on page 66. The cats and dogs serve in this case to balance your back muscles out after a rotation and to restore functional glide between your arm bones and shoulder blades.

KNEELING WALL CLOCK
Duration: 1 minute each position

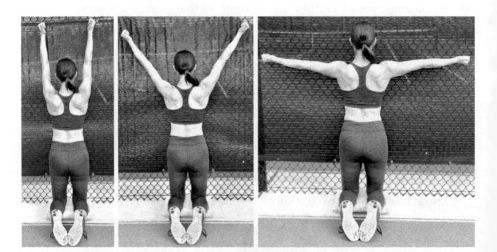

There are three positions held for one minute each. If any position creates pain, skip it for now and go to the next one. After a few days or weeks, you'll be able to come back to it and it should feel better. You'll start kneeling with your knees touching the wall, feet pigeon-toed and arms straight up overhead. Lock out your elbows, make a fist with your thumbs up and rotate out from your shoulder, pulling your thumbs away from the wall. After a minute, drop your arms out to 45 degrees for another minute, then to 90 degrees for the final minute. Not only is this exercise realigning your entire upper back, but it's also strengthening the movers and powerful stabilizers of your shoulders.

Wrist Pain

Wrist pain and injury always stems from a rotational issue with the bones of the forearm, which is correlated with the function of the shoulder. In other words, your wrist pain is always a sign of misalignment of the elbow and arm bones.

The wrist, in addition to being able to rotate, also flexes and extends laterally and from front to back. During tennis, your wrist is put in a position of extreme extension during a forehand and slight flexion on the backhand, and it's the first point of contact to absorb the force transmitted from your racket to your arm. The wrist and ankle are similar that way in that the ankle is the first major joint to absorb the force of contact with the ground.

Thus, there is a somewhat similar design and function to them both (after all, we probably crawled on all fours at one point in time).

Again, do these exercises in the order they appear and never push through pain. The exercises for the elbow and shoulder can also serve to cure your wrist pain, but start with these:

AB CRUNCHES
Repetitions: 50

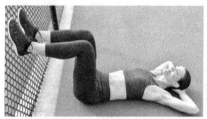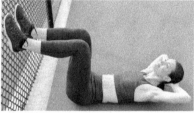

With your feet on the wall and knees bent 90 degrees, interlace your fingers together behind your head. Keep your elbows back as you raise your upper body off the ground about six inches. Keep your head back and your elbows pulled back as you rise up off the ground. DON'T CURL YOUR ELBOWS FORWARD OR BRING YOUR CHIN Toward YOUR CHEST. Instead, pull your upper body straight up toward the sky. It helps to keep your eyes fixed on something behind you as you come up so your head doesn't come forward. This exercise isn't for your stomach, although that's where you'll feel it. It's resetting the functional alignment between your shoulder blades, shoulder joint, elbow and wrist. As you come up, it provides a distraction (pulling away) force to your wrist joint. That is, as long as you keep your elbows pulled back as your upper body raises up.

CROCODILE

See the instructions earlier in this chapter. The purpose of the crocodile in this case is to remind your wrist, elbow and shoulder joint to rotate together as a unit.

PELVIC TILTS
Repetitions: 10

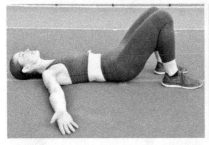 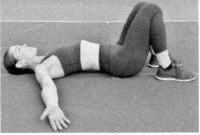

Lying on your back with your knees bent and feet flat on the ground, press your lower back flat into the ground until there's no space. Next, roll your hips forward toward your knees to induce an arch in your low back. Roll back and forth, keeping your butt on the ground the entire time. The purpose of the pelvic tilts is to restore proper motion to your hips and your lumbar spine.

STATIC BACK PULLOVERS
Repetitions: 30

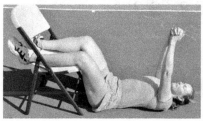 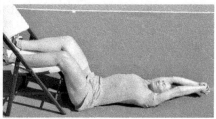

Lie on your back with your knees up on a chair, ottoman or couch. Your hips should be up to the chair, and your knees and hips as close to 90 degrees as you can get them. Interlace your fingers, with your palms touching, and pull your arms straight up overhead, keeping your elbows locked and arms straight. Try to touch the ground overhead if you can; otherwise, go as far as you can and then return to the starting position. This is a key exercise to restore motion and function to your shoulder joint. As your shoulder restores its proper function and alignment, your wrist will stop compensating and the pain can diminish.

CHAPTER 23

HIPS AND MOBILITY

L ike most sports, tennis is almost entirely driven by the hips, which provide balance, mobility, and power. Good hip function not only gets you to the ball quickly and efficiently, but also keeps you from falling over once you get there. Hip mobility and stability are also imperative to helping with shoulder turn and your ability to transfer your weight correctly to your front foot on a groundstroke. In other words, they're essential to everything. If you want to play your best tennis, you have to have functional hips.

The good news is that improving your hip function even a little will improve your movement, and your game, by a lot.

Good mobility provides the ultimate advantage on the tennis court. It evens the playing field at all levels, but especially as you get older. After all, it doesn't matter how well you hit the ball if you can't get to it. Every day, players of lesser ability beat better hitters because they can get to more balls, and thus hit more balls back in the court. Tennis is a sport won or lost on errors, not winners, so getting more balls in play almost always translates to winning.

Obviously, if you have any kind of pain in your hips, you're probably not feeling that mobile, so the first step will be to eliminate any nagging ailments.

Before you jump into the exercises, though, let's revisit three quick assessments to provide a basic understanding of what's contributing to or causing the pain:

1. As you look at your hips in the mirror does one look higher or closer to you?
2. When you look down at your feet is one foot in front of the other?
3. Close your eyes and feel your weight distribution. Is there more weight on one leg?

Remember, the painful hip is very often the one that is overloaded and working the hardest, which is why it hurts.

These positional clues are all signs of imbalanced and misaligned hips. The pain itself is a clue as to specifically where your hip is being overworked and overstressed. That's why you can often solve the pain by changing the position of the hips. By realigning the joint, you immediately decrease the amount of pressure and stress on your hip, which allows damaged joint and muscle tissue to heal.

As you'll also recall from earlier chapters, anytime your hips are off there is automatically an imbalance in your spinal muscles that run from your lower back all the way to your neck. The resulting disparity in tension in your shoulder blades leads to one shoulder blade looking and functioning differently from the other.

This interconnectedness between all the body's parts dictates the need to treat the body as a unit. Therefore, by addressing your shoulder imbalance and function you will immediately impact and improve your hip imbalance and function, and vice versa.

This hip restoration routine will take you anywhere from thirty minutes to an hour. The extra time is due to the supine groin stretch exercise, which should be done a minimum of fifteen minutes per side. This is a key exercise to reset your hip joint and your spine back to neutral, which takes some time as the layers of compensating muscles begin to relax and let go. As always, do these exercises in the order they appear and skip anything that increases pain for now.

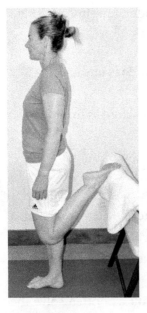

STANDING QUAD STRETCH
Duration: 1 minute

This exercise restores proper function to the hip joint while reminding your upper body to remain evenly centered over your hips. Put one leg behind you on a chair or table keeping your knees level (when you look down one knee should not be in front of the other). Tuck your hips under by rolling your pelvis down toward your heels. Try not to shift your hips forward like you're doing a standing backbend. If you need to hold on to a wall or a chair for balance, go ahead, but don't lean on the wall. Focus on keeping your hips level as you stand rather than letting the standing leg shift out.

SUPINE GROIN STRETCH
Duration: 15 to 30 minutes per side

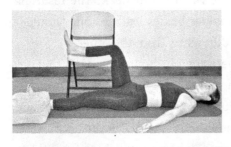

Lie on your back with one leg up on a chair at 90 degrees and the other leg on the ground in line with your hip (not out to the side). Prop something up against your outer ankle on the down leg so the foot stays pointing straight up toward the ceiling without you having to hold it there. Relax your arms out to your sides with your palms up and breathe. There should be no tension anywhere in your body. This is the one exercise that will realign your hip joint one at a time without your body being able to cheat, twist, turn or compensate. Time is truly your best friend here because this exercise asks the groin muscles, hip flexors and deep hip rotators to balance out with your spinal muscles. Use the *thigh test* to determine how much is enough by contracting the muscles on the front of your thigh when you first get into the exercise, again in five minutes, and again after fifteen minutes. Don't hold the contraction. Squeeze the thigh muscles for two seconds then let go just to establish where the muscle contracts. At first, you'll feel most of the contraction toward your knee. Over time, you'll feel it move up the thigh until it gets into your hip. You'll know you're cooked when you contract your thigh muscles and you feel the entire thigh contract rather than just the muscles close to your knee.

FLOOR BLOCK
Duration: 1 minute each position

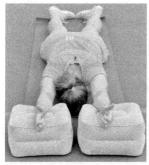 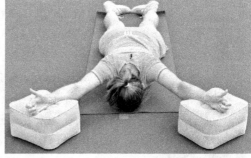

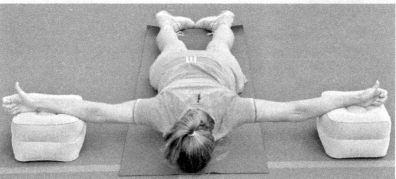

Hip misalignment is synonymous with shoulder misalignment, so you need to address both considering your shoulders and hips are connected to the same spine. This is a great exercise to balance out your spinal muscles top to bottom, right to left and to ultimately reposition your hips. Lie on your stomach with forehead on the ground and place your arms straight above your head with each forearm on a pillow. You can use pillows from your bed or couch, yoga blocks, or stack some books about six inches. Lock out your elbows, pigeon-toe your feet with your heels dropped out and make a fist with your thumbs up. Rotate your thumbs up toward the sky like you're trying to point them behind you.

AIRBENCH
Duration: 1 to 2 minutes

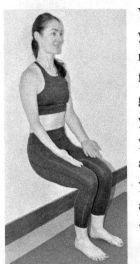

You'll finish off with the airbench to make sure your hips are balanced right to left and to mitigate any rotation in your lower back. You'll feel your quads fatigue quickly, but they'll grow stronger with a little practice. Make sure you press your lower back into the wall, drop your hips to just above 90 degrees, keep your ankles directly under, or slightly in front, of your knees. Your feet should point straight ahead and should be about one to two fist-widths apart.

Make sure to test your weight distribution, your hip rotation and your foot position again after the exercises. You should notice a change not only in how your hips feel but also in how you look. Do this hip routine every day for up to two weeks if needed and then do it from time to time as desired just to keep things balanced.

CHAPTER 24

RESILIENT KNEES

K nees are the less mobile but very stable counterparts to the extremely mobile ankle and hip joints. While the ankles and hips move from side to side and rotate in and out, the knees are supposed to only bend and straighten. They move in one plane of motion while the hips and ankles move in many ways and have several functions.

The knees are also designed to have balanced muscle tension on all sides to allow for fluid motion and for the knee to be neutrally aligned. However, there are conditions in which the knees aren't stressed equally on both sides and the flexion and extension functions don't work optimally.

For example, *knock knees* or *bowlegs* are familiar terms and common traits. With both, knee alignment is greatly altered in relation to the joints above and below the knee (Figs. *24.1* and *24.2* below). In the case of bowlegs (technically called *varus stress*), the knee is aligned to the outside in relation to the hip joint. In people with knock knees (*valgus stress*), the knee is aligned toward the inside of the hip joint.

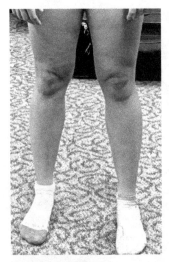 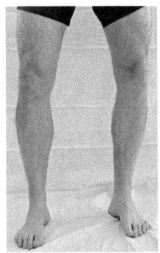

Figure 24.1 Valgus stress   *Figure 24.2 Varus stress*

In either case, the knee is no longer aligned directly under the hip joint, which means the bones that make up the knee (the femur and tibia) are no longer in their balanced and neutral positions. Since these bones don't line up correctly, the consequence is uneven wear and tear on the cartilage, which often leads to early and sometimes complete deterioration of the tissue. Eventually for many, the joint can become bone on bone.

My stepfather was a prime example. He was so bowlegged that even just standing still it looked like he was still riding a horse. He waddled when he walked because his knee wasn't bending properly due to the bow, and eventually because of the pain.

As I've always said, there's a time and a place for surgery, and by that point his knees (and more importantly, his pain) seemed to be beyond non-surgical help.

The result was a double knee replacement. The good news is he feels much better and that was the right choice for him.

Despite my stepdad's situation, the knees are incredibly resilient joints, which makes it possible for many people to get out of pain non-surgically. If you catch it early enough, are ready to put in the work, and you start before the cartilage is all gone, you have a chance of getting by with good therapy. Even in the case of bone on bone (total cartilage loss in one spot), by aligning the knee with the right exercises the pain can often be greatly diminished.

No matter what state your knee is in, though, there's absolutely no downside to starting the exercises now. (This is where you feel my elbow nudging you in the side).

Meniscus Tears

The most common knee symptoms in tennis players include pain on the inside or outside of the knee, meniscus tears, and patellar tendonitis. Pain on the either side of the knee and meniscus tears (tears in the cartilage) are common with all misalignments of the knee. The meniscus, which acts as the major shock absorber of the knee, tears when load and torque is added to a misaligned knee. In tennis, it usually happens when someone plants and then turns suddenly while that leg is still planted. The result is a sheer force that literally tears the tissue.

Of course, the problem wasn't the plant and turn; you've done that a million times before without tearing anything. The issue was the plant and turn on a knee that wasn't aligned, and the compensating muscles were already worn down as a result of fatigue. In other words, it was an accident waiting to happen.

If you have a torn meniscus or pain in the inside or outside of your knee, these exercises will help realign and rebalance the muscles from your ankle to your hip and beyond.

Time: 5 minutes, 1 to 2 times per day

FLEXION AB POSITION
Duration: 3 minutes

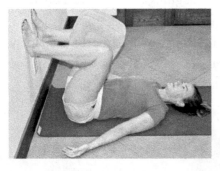

Lie on your back with your feet on the wall and your hips six to eight inches away from the wall. Your lower legs should be parallel to the floor and your feet straight. Squeeze a pillow between your knees and hold. Relax your shoulders and focus on making the squeeze even between both inner thighs. You might feel like the inner thigh of the hurt knee is working less or differently, so wait it out until both legs feel even and equal even if it goes beyond three minutes. Keep your feet pointing straight up the wall and squeeze hard. This is a great exercise to wake up the powerful hip and thigh muscles that support your knee and to realign your upper and lower leg bones that make up the knee joint.

STATIC WALL PULLBACKS
Repetitions: 3 sets of 10 each leg

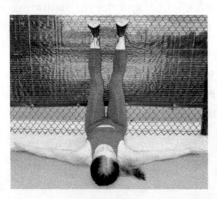

Lie on your back with your legs up a wall. Your feet should be about the width of your fist apart. Push your knees toward the wall, flex your feet back toward your knees, place your palms up out to the sides and contract your thigh muscles. Keeping the knee locked and thigh tight, pull one heel off the wall up and down ten times, then switch legs. Make sure your knee doesn't bend, your hips stay on the ground, and you keep your foot straight the whole time. This exercise engages the prime movers and stabilizers of the knee and hip and retrains the leg to work as a unit.

SITTING STATIC KNEE PILLOW SQUEEZE
Duration: 2 minutes

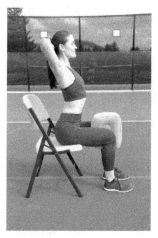

This one will make you sweat, so be ready. Sit toward the middle of the chair with your hips rolled forward to create an arch in your lower back. Keep your feet straight and your ankles directly under your knees to form a right angle between your lower and upper legs. Interlace your fingers behind your head and pull your elbows back as far as you can. Use a pillow from your bed or couch or a yoga block between your knees and squeeze hard and hold. Again, you're waiting until both inner thighs are working evenly, but no matter what, hold at least two minutes or until the work is balanced. Oh, and don't forget to smile. This exercise will even up the workload in your hips and engage all the powerful movers and stabilizers of your hips and knees while taking your upper back completely out of play.

Patellar Tendonitis

The patellar tendon is more of a ligament. It connects the patella, the circular bony part on the front of your knee, to the shin bone, and it works to keep the patella in place while helping the quadriceps straighten the leg. It also helps to keep the upper leg bone, the femur, from sliding forward over the lower leg bone, the tibia.

Patellar tendonitis, or pain on the front of the knee, is often the result of too much force on the front of the knee due to misaligned hips and rotation in the knee joint. You can usually predict it by looking at your side-view pictures. When the hip joint is forward of the knee from the side view, the center of gravity has moved forward with it. Instead of the stress of gravity going through the middle of your knee, it's now displaced, towing the front directly over the tendon. The pain is a response to the overloaded and stressed patellar tendon, which is being forced to bear the lion's share of the body weight while also desperately trying to keep the femur from sliding forward over the tibia.

A rotation of the hips toward one side can also have the same effect of displacing the center of gravity forward over the patellar tendon while also adding an extra torque to the knee joint as well.

Traditional therapy works to strengthen the quadriceps muscles, which implies they're weak. There's a major problem with that assessment though. Since the pain is usually only in one knee and shows up unannounced one day, how did those muscles suddenly become weak over the course of a day? They don't.

A better explanation is the pelvis rotated or moved forward of the ankles just enough to inhibit the quad muscles from firing. *Muscle inhibition* is a term describing the inability of a muscle to fire because the joint is out of position. It has nothing to do with weakness.

We're going to treat the condition a little differently than the traditional approach. Whether both hips are forward, or just one, the goal is the same in terms of fixing the real problem. Align the hips over the ankles. You have to take the torque out of the knee, and you have to get the knee joint acting as a hinge again. Once you do that, your patellar tendon will be extremely grateful and will love you forever.

As usual, do these exercises exactly in the order they appear and skip anything that causes pain.

Time: 7 minutes 1 to 2 times per day.

FLEXION ABS
Repetitions: 2x25 (50 total)

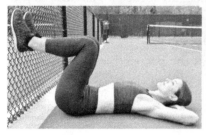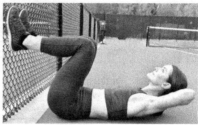

With your feet on the wall pointing straight up and knees bent to 45 degrees, interlace your fingers behind your head and pull your elbows back toward the ground. Crunch up by bringing your upper body six to eight inches off the floor, but keep your elbows pulled back and look behind you as you rise. It helps to squeeze a pillow between your knees as you do this exercise to keep even tension in your hips. The goal is to engage the deep hip flexors, which stabilize the hip and, consequently, the knee considering the hip joint and the knee joint share the same leg bone (the femur).

FLEXION AB HAMSTRING GLIDES
Repetitions: 3x10 (30 total)

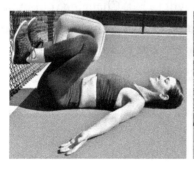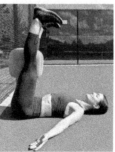

In the same position as the flexion abs before, place a pillow between your knees and squeeze hard. Keep your feet and ankles flexed back toward your knees as you pull your feet off the wall and drop your heels toward the ground without touching the wall. Then straighten up your legs in the air until your knees are locked (or as close as you can get to it). Repeat ten times, then rest.

Relax your upper body the entire time and let your hips and legs do the work. This exercise restores the proper glide in your knee joint while isolating the major movers and stabilizers of your hips and knees.

STATIC EXTENSION
Duration: 2 minutes

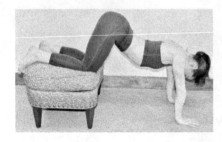

Place your knees on an ottoman, low couch or chair and your hands on the ground. Walk your hands forward until your hips are no more than six to eight inches ahead of your knees. Your hands should be directly under your shoulders with your elbows locked. Let your back sway, your shoulder blades drop together and your head drop. This is a fantastic exercise to realign your hips with your mid and upper back and to balance out your body from right to left. Changing your upper body alignment will redirect the stress of gravity through your knees.

Do the exercises specific to your condition every day for one to three weeks. You'll find out as you go that your knees won't be the only joints that feel better. But I'll let you discover the other accompanying benefits for yourself.

CHAPTER 25

STABLE ANKLES AND HAPPY FEET

E very tennis player deals with foot or ankle issues at some time in their career.

My first memorable run-in with foot pain came in the semifinals of the Junior Intermountain 18s sectionals, the last sectional tournament before the junior summer national series.

I was playing my good friend and doubles partner when I ran for a ball and felt a slight twinge of pain on the top of my foot. It didn't stop me from continuing, but the next morning I could barely walk. I learned a few days later I had a stress fracture in my foot. Thinking my worn-out shoes were to blame, I gave it three weeks to heal and went back to playing.

My next painful encounter occurred during my freshman year at UC Berkeley. I was walking back to my dorm after team practice one afternoon and a sharp pain in my ankle dropped me to the ground like I'd been stabbed by an ice pick. I learned via X-ray I was the not-so-proud owner of a rather large bone spur on the outer part of my ankle joint.

Nobody knew how a bone spur magically appeared on the same foot and ankle I had stress fractured a year earlier, so I had surgery to remove it, and again blamed my shoes.

My last incident happened during a tour of minor pro tournaments in Mexico—a four-tournament satellite circuit. The first tournament was on red clay that was so slippery it was like playing hockey with a tennis racket. As many of you who have played on clay know, sliding on a clay court is common and often necessary to get to the ball, especially on a slippery court where footing is difficult.

Ironically, the culprit wasn't the slippery clay, or the slide, it was the hard-court tournament that followed. During my first practice on the hard-court in preparation for the next tournament, I ran for a wide ball to my forehand, planted too early like I was going to slide, and folded my ankle over like it was paper origami. I didn't walk for a week without crutches and didn't walk normally for another three weeks after that.

In truth, ankle origami was common for me; I rolled my ankle about every few weeks to the point where my ligaments were so stretched out it didn't even bother me anymore.

Why am I telling you all this? Because there were three separate incidences, all seemingly unrelated, all from the same underlying cause. It wasn't the shoes, or the tennis court, or the fact that I'm just a tennis player and that's how it goes. The cause was my imbalanced right hip and the position of my right ankle.

I was bringing an ankle that was already rolled outward (supinated) to every tennis court I played on, no matter the surface. It was rolled to the outside instead of being more neutral because of a tight right hip flexor and an equally tight right glute muscle that had rotated my knee out, which rolled my foot toward the outside edge along with it.

The technical term is *supination* with the result being constant strain on the outside muscles, bones, ligaments, and tendons on my foot and ankle. You can see it and feel it for yourself if you stand up and roll to the outside of your feet.

Watch your arches come way up and your knees rotate out as you do it. In my case, it was coming from the hip down rather than from the ankle up, but the result is the same—an ankle or foot injury waiting to happen.

Of course, there's always an incident that makes it appear as if it's a traumatic injury, but my joint was already compromised and vulnerable to the slightest overload or stress. All of this due to the imbalanced muscles and alignment of my hip, knee and ankle.

At the time, the well-meaning doctors, trainers, and therapists that helped me recover from the stress fracture, bone spur, and ankle sprain never thought to check my foot position, or considered my hip tightness. Plus, we all blamed the shoes, or tennis, or plain old bad luck. Now I know better. And now you do, too.

Most injuries don't just happen for random reasons. They're clues as to where your body is being stressed due to an imbalance and misalignment somewhere along the musculoskeletal chain. Remember, we bend or break at our weakest points. Your job is to discover where those weak points are and to fix the underlying imbalances behind them.

Here are some common foot ailments tennis players face, along with some common causes, and the exercise sets to address them:

Plantar fasciitis and Achilles Tendonitis

I group these symptoms together because irritation of the fascia on the foot and Achilles tendonitis often go together with the same posture. Plantar fasciitis is the painful inflammation of the connective tissue on the bottom of your foot, and Achilles tendonitis is the inflammation of the tendon on the back of your heel. Traditional therapy blames tight calf and hamstring muscles for both. But what's causing the tightness?

Usually, the painful condition on one foot is an indication your hip, knee, and ankle are all bearing too much of the body weight compared to the other side, and your body is pitching forward on both sides, or on one side, from the side view (Fig. *25.1*). The term *pitching forward* describes when the hip and shoulder joints are in front of the ankle joint in your side view pictures.

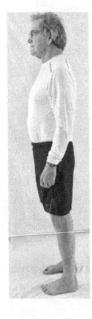

Figure 25.1 Notice the entire body sitting forward of the ankles.

As your body leans forward, your hamstrings, back muscles, calf muscles, Achilles, and muscles in the arch of your foot grab on for dear life to keep you from falling on your face. Couple that with the overload on that foot, and you have too much stress on the muscles and fascia of the foot, and on the Achilles tendon. Therefore, you have to change the posture to change the pressure.

Time: 10 to 12 minutes 1 to 3 times/day until the pain abates

Counter Stretch
Duration: 1 minute

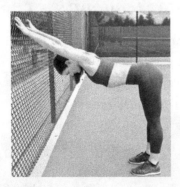

Place your hands on a wall, walk your feet back and bend at the waist as low as you can comfortably go without stressing your shoulders. Your ankles should be directly below your hips. Create an arch in your low back by rolling your hips forward from the front of your hip bones and let your back sway. Contract your thigh muscles and make sure your feet are pointing straight ahead and six inches apart. This exercise engages and reconnects the entire backside of your body while repositioning your upper back.

HIP LIFT WITH FOOT CIRCLES POINT FLEXES
Repetitions: 20 foot circles each direction and 20 point flexes

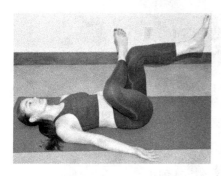

While on your back with your palms up out to your sides, cross one ankle over the other knee. Raise the bottom leg to 90 degrees at the hip and the knee. Use your leg muscles to push the crossed leg away from you as you keep the other knee still.

Circle the uncrossed ankle and foot twenty times in each direction, then pull the foot back all the way followed by pointing it twenty times. Switch sides by crossing the opposite ankle over the knee and repeat. Don't use your hands to hold your knees up! Relax your arms at your sides AT ALL TIMES. We want your hip muscles doing the work, not your upper body. This exercise kills two birds with one stone as it realigns the hips with the upper body and restores strength and motion to all the muscles of the feet and ankles.

KNEELING GROIN STRETCH
Duration: 1 minute

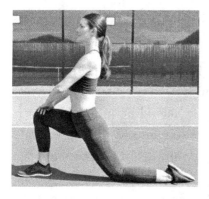

With one knee on the ground lunge forward with the other leg while dropping your hips down toward the ground until you feel a stretch on the front of your thigh. Keep your upper body straight and your front foot pointing straight ahead. This exercise reminds your hip joint of its full range of motion instead of stopping too early and letting your calf muscles take over.

ASSISTED RUNNER'S STRETCH
Duration 1 minute each side

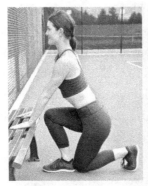 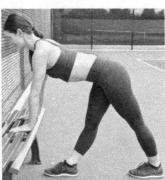

Begin by kneeling on one knee with your hands on a chair or couch and your back knee touching your front heel. Keeping your hands on the chair, stand up until both legs are straight with your knees locked out and your heels on the ground. Try to roll your hips forward to create a slight arch in your low back. You'll feel the increased stretch on the back of your leg as you do. This exercise connects all the muscles of the back of your leg, including the calves and hamstrings, and it reminds your hips they're designed to fully flex and extend rather than rotate.

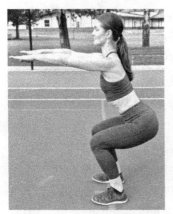

WIDE FREE SQUAT
Duration: 1 minute

Squat from a standing position until your hips are just above your knees. Your feet should be hip-width apart, your feet straight and your upper body as straight and upright as possible. Your arms and hands should be parallel to the ground. The squat engages your glutes (butt muscles), hamstrings (the muscles on the back of your thighs) and your thigh muscles. It also balances your weight distribution between hips while repositioning your upper body.

Ankle Sprain/Pain

Ankle sprains are no fun, but heal very quickly with the right stimulus. What I didn't mention in my story above was that as soon as I started doing the exercises to realign my ankle, knee, and hip, I never sprained my ankle again. What used to be a common, nagging occurrence completely disappeared like a mosquito in the wind.

The key is to take the rotation out of the ankle joint, and to get the ankle, knee and hip working together as a unit again with all the stabilizing muscles doing their jobs.

As always, do the exercises in the order they appear and never push through pain. If an exercise incites pain, then skip it for now and try it again in two to three days.

ELEVATED LYING SUPINE FEET TIED
Duration: 7 minutes per level for 3 levels

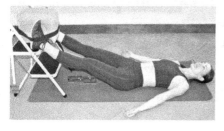

While lying on your back and with your shoes on, place your heels on the edge of a stepladder or stepping stool. Your feet will have a pillow between them, and a belt or yoga strap tied around the outsides of your feet to keep your feet pointing straight up and slightly pulled back toward your knees without having to consciously hold that position. Relax your arms out to the sides with your palms up. After seven minutes drop your heels one level down, again placing them on the edge of the ladder. Drop your heels every seven minutes to a lower level with the last level as the one just above the floor. You should try to get at least three levels, including the last. This exercise takes the torque out of the ankle and realigns it with the knee and the hip joint. Time is your best friend on this one, so don't get antsy and come up early.

Static Wall Femur Rotations
Sets and Repetitions: 15 rotations in and out in 3 positions (45 rotations total)

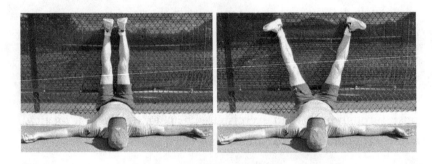

Lie on your back with your legs straight up the wall. Tighten your thighs while pushing your knees toward the wall to take out any bend in the knee. Flex your feet back toward you, keeping your feet straight. With your legs hip-width apart rotate your legs in and out (rotating from the hip joint) without letting the knees bend. After fifteen reps spread your legs to 45 degrees and repeat, then again with your legs spread slightly wider. Relax your upper body entirely. This exercise wakes up the hip muscles, which are often shut off after an ankle sprain.

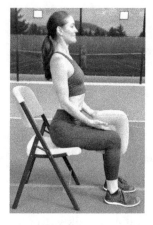

SITTING KNEE PILLOW SQUEEZES
Repetitions: 60

Sit toward the middle of a chair with your ankles directly under your knees and your hips rolled forward to create an arch in your low back. Place a pillow from your bed or couch (or a yoga block will do) and squeeze and release. Keep your feet straight and slightly less than hip-width apart. This exercise will remind your ankles, knees and hips to work together again and to bear balanced weight.

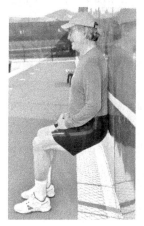

AIRBENCH
Duration: 1 minute

Skip this exercise if there's too much pain still to put weight on the ankle that's sprained; otherwise, slide your hips down the wall to just above 90 degrees, press your low back flat into the wall and keep your feet pointing straight ahead. Your ankles should be slightly forward or directly under your knees and about a fist-width apart. Either way, you should be able to see your toes. The airbench repositions the ankle back to neutral and reconnects the muscles from the ankle all the way to the hip.

Bunions

Aside from tight shoes pushing your big toe over and squishing your feet, bunions also come from your foot turning out rather than pointing straight ahead. The result is when your foot trails behind you in normal walking, called *toe off*, you end up pushing all your weight off of the inside of your big toe rather than off all five toes equally. The bunion is essentially a buildup of tissue, like a callous forming on your foot, as your body's natural reaction to an overload of stress in that area.

To illustrate the cause of the bunion, stand and walk with one foot turned out. You'll notice you now hit on the outside of your heel and foot first rather than directly on the heel, and your foot rolls from outside to inside as it accepts the weight. Also, notice that as you push off your foot, you push off from the inside of your big toe—exactly where the bunion is.

Once you use the exercises to change the position of your foot to point more straight ahead, the stress on that spot will be relieved, and the bunion can diminish and eventually disappear. It's no different than a callous that would vanish from your racket hand if you were to stop playing tennis.

The first step to curing your bunions is to make sure you have shoes wide enough to allow your toes to spread. In other words, don't wear shoes that squish your toes. I also recommend wearing toe spacers from time to time, which accomplish the same goal. The next step is to reposition your foot and to reconnect it to your ankle, knee and hip, which is what the exercises are designed to do below. The routine will take you five minutes.

SUPINE FOOT CIRCLES POINT FLEXES
Repetitions: 40 circles each direction followed by 40 point/flexes

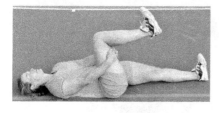

You'll be surprised how quickly your ankles and shins will fatigue at first as this exercise wakes up all the muscles of your foot and ankle and reminds them of their full range of motion and function. Begin by lying on your back and interlacing your hands under one knee while straightening out the opposite leg on the ground. Keep your shoulders relaxed down and back and the foot of the straight leg pointed toward the sky. Circle the foot of your bent knee one direction forty times, making as full a circle as you can, then switch directions. Once the circles are complete, point and flex your foot back and forth.

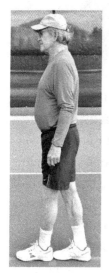

IN-LINE GLUTE CONTRACTIONS
Repetitions: 20 each leg, repeat 3x

Stand with your feet touching and in-line, with the toes of one foot touching the heel of the other. Unlike the model in the picture who had to wear shoes because the court was too hot, do this exercise in bare feet. Keep your weight even on both feet and your legs straight as you squeeze and release your butt muscles. Relax your shoulders and keep your upper body straight. Once you've hit twenty reps put the other leg in front and repeat. Go back and forth every twenty reps until you've completed three sets. This exercise reminds your body what it's like when your foot, knee and hip point in the same direction while asking the key balancing muscles of your feet and ankle to work overtime and do their jobs.

FLOOR BLOCK
Duration: 1 minute each position

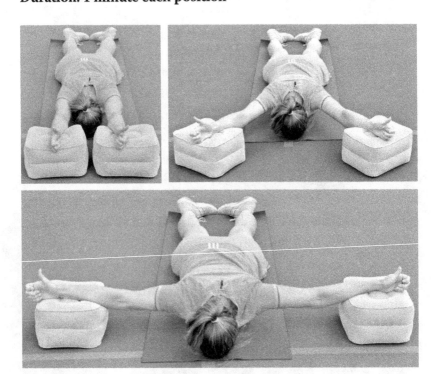

Lie down on your stomach with your forehead on the ground (use a towel or a mat as a cushion). Touch your toes together and allow your heels to drop away from each other. Place your arms on yoga blocks, stacked books or pillows about six inches high, just below your elbows or around the middle of your forearms. Don't worry if the block or pillow height isn't exact. Lock out your elbows, make a fist with your thumbs up and rotate your thumbs up toward the sky. Hold a minute, then bring the blocks and your arms out to 45 degrees and repeat, then 90 degrees. The body is a unit, so by changing the position of your upper body you'll change the function of your hips and, consequently, the stress and position of your feet.

Keeping Your Feet Healthy and Happy

No matter what your feet look like—pretty or pretty ugly—I have some tips for happy feet. Happy feet usually translate to a happy body, so it's important to be kind to them.

Our feet are our first contact with the environment. They're the soldiers on the ground (pun intended) that relay information to the brain about our terrain. The brain then sends commands back to the muscles and joints in our feet to provide balance and coordination while standing and walking.

When we wear shoes, those messages get diluted because the shoes make first contact with the ground rather than the soles of our feet. Therefore, our brain responds to the contortions of the shoe first, which usually doesn't contort much at all, and any normal shoe is extremely rigid compared to your very mobile and pliable foot.

Shoes then become like casts for our feet because they limit the motion of the foot. The stiffer the shoe, the harder the cast. Rather than the joints and muscles going through a full range of motion while walking and absorbing the rich and varied stimulus they're designed to receive, they only get the stimulus the shoe allows. Unfortunately, our feet are worse off for it as the muscles and joints become weaker due to the lack of stimulation.

Happy, healthy feet require lots of stimulation and a little love, and they'll repay you by carrying you to the next drop shot without complaint.

My seven tips for happy feet:

1. Take your shoes off and walk barefoot as often as possible.
2. Walk in sand. Walking in sand is great for strengthening your feet, and sand helps to wake up all the muscles in the arch of your foot and ankle.

3. Spread your toes—literally—from time to time with your fingers or work on doing it with your toe and foot muscles. There are also shoes that will help to keep your toes spread. I recommend the FiveFinger shoes from Vibram, which spread your toes and allow all five digits to get in on the action. If those aren't your thing (they feel goofy at first), then there are many other barefoot brands that are light and roomy and allow your foot some freedom. Investing in some toe spacers also wouldn't be a bad idea.

4. If your feet hurt, try to wear a less bulky and rigid shoe, as opposed to more supportive, as often as you can. The more the shoe compensates for your lack of foot strength and function, the weaker you'll get, and the more dependent you'll be on the shoe in the short and the long run.

5. Pick tennis shoes that are the most comfortable to you. Don't pick the ones the shoe salesman picked for you, or the most popular brand. Wear the ones that feel the best. Period. If you have a choice, I personally prefer lighter tennis shoes to heavier ones, and wider shoes compared to more narrow ones, which allow more space and freedom for your feet.

6. Clip your toe nails. There are few things more painful than jamming a toe nail while playing tennis. I've seen people default matches for this very reason, so keep your nails short.

7. Get foot rubs often. Massages are good for your feet, they stimulate meridian lines throughout your body, they feel amazing, and you could use a break anyway!

Remember, our feet evolved over millions of years to be without shoes like every other animal on the planet. Other than using them for protection against nails and glass and other sharp objects in the concrete jungle we live in, we don't technically need them; we've just gotten used to wearing them.

PART V

THE NEW YOU

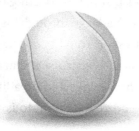

CHAPTER 26

RELIABLE RITUALS

I want you to repeatedly experience tennis-winning bliss rather than crappy-play-provoking grief. And I want you to feel great while doing it. Therefore, I've created one quick pre-tennis routine before you play, and a post-tennis routine.

Every pro uses reliable and familiar routines and rituals in competition to help them focus and to cope with pressure. They do it to make everything automatic and to eliminate the variables so they can focus on the task at hand—beating the other player.

We've all seen Rafael Nadal go through his rituals of touching his face and ears, picking his shorts out of crevices, and turning his water bottles to face the outside. We also see Sharapova turn away from the baseline to pick at her strings and do a little jog before serving or returning. What we don't see them do is warm up their bodies before going on the court.

I assure you, they have a consistent, reliable routine they do *every* time, just like the rituals they follow on the court, so they can be ready to go from the first point. Once they find a routine that works for them, it's one less thing to worry about, as well as one more variable they can somewhat control—how their body feels before facing their opponent.

You can do a bunch of different random stretches or exercises (or nothing) before you play, but then you leave how you feel up to chance. One day you might feel great and play great, the next day you might feel stiff and take a set to get going, or maybe you never get going at all. We've all had those days. In fact, it happens to most amateur players and some pros more often than it should.

Pre-Tennis Warm-Up

This pre-tennis routine will prepare you mentally and physically to bring out your best from the first ball to the last. The ultimate goal here is not just to warm you up; it's to prevent injury, to bring your body to neutral and balanced, to prime your body for the upcoming physical demand, to put you in a position to play your best tennis, and to further your goal of playing as much tennis as you want for as long as you want, no matter what your age.

If you're doing a specific stroke menu from the Tennis Commandment chapter, do that first, then do your pre-tennis routine.

Do these exercises *exactly* in the order they appear because there's a method to the saneness. Each exercise prepares you for the next and is a progression in demand and function. These exercises are specifically chosen to:

1. Activate and align all the major load joints.
2. Prepare your hips and spine for rotation as well as flexion and extension.
3. Engage your wrist, elbow and shoulders to prepare them for battle.
4. Remind your body to work together as a unit.

The routine will take you ten minutes and can be done on or off the court. You can watch the video instructions of each exercise in the pre and post tennis routines at www.egoscue.com/agelesstennis.

Standing Arm Circles
Repetitions: 40 palms down forward, 40 palms up backward

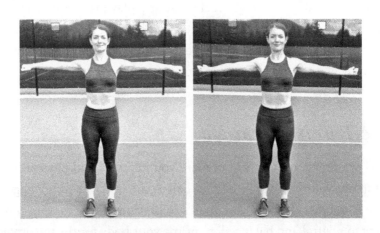

Stand with your feet straight, your arms straight out from your shoulders and your shoulder blades squeezed together. Think of pulling your shoulders down and back away from your ears. Make what we call a golfer's grip with your hands where you spread your fingers out, then curl the top knuckles tight into the palms of your hands. Keep your feet pointing straight ahead and about six to eight inches apart. Relax your stomach. With your thumbs pointing straight ahead make small circles at a medium pace in the direction of your thumb. To be clear, begin by circling up and in the direction of your thumb. Do forty circles, and then rotate your palms up keeping the same grip and do forty circles backward.

Imagine doing circles around your own fist and that's how big the circles will be. The arm circles not only warm up your arms and shoulders, they also begin to realign your upper back along with all your load joints.

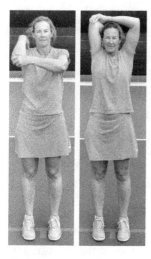

TRICEPS STRETCH
Duration: 1 minute each side

In a standing position with your feet pointing straight ahead, place one hand on the same shoulder and the opposite hand on that elbow. Keeping your hand on your shoulder, bring that elbow straight up and back. Relax your stomach and feel the slight stretch in your shoulder. Allow the opposite arm to come up overhead as it holds your elbow. This exercise is engaging the extensors of your spine, balancing your hips out from right to left, and preparing your shoulders for overhead motion.

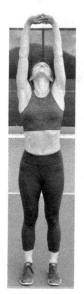

STANDING OVERHEAD EXTENSION
Duration: 1 minute

Stand with your feet straight six inches apart. Interlace your fingers together and turn your palms away from you. Bring your hands straight up overhead while locking out your elbows. Pull back as far as you can and reach for the sky. Don't let your hips shift forward like you're in a backbend. Instead, keep your hips over your heels. Look up toward your hands, relax your stomach and hold. This exercise engages all the muscles on the back side of your body from heel to head to get them ready to go, and it realigns your upper back, shoulders and hips to a more neutral position.

HIP CROSSOVER STRETCH
Duration: 1 minute each side

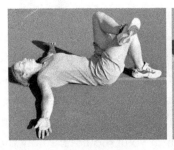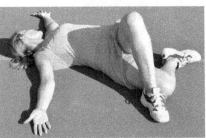

Lie on your back and bend both knees. Cross one ankle over the other knee and drop that foot over to the opposite side until the outside of the down leg is on the ground and the foot is flat. Use your leg muscles (not your hands) to push the knee that's pointing toward the sky away from you. You will feel a stretch in the outside of your hip or leg. The hip crossover stretch reduces any hip imbalance and rotation and engages the lateral hip muscles, which you'll need when moving from side to side.

CATS AND DOGS
Repetitions: 10 cats and 10 dogs

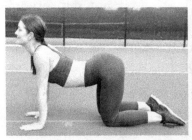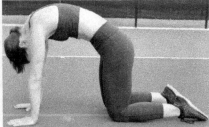

Go on your hands and knees with your hands directly under your shoulders and your knees directly under your hips. Let your back drop and your shoulder blades come together, but initiate the movement from your hips not your spine. Look up as your back drops. Reverse directions by using your hips to begin to round your back up toward the sky and drop your head. This exercise brings the muscles on the front and backside of your body back to balance.

Downward Dog to Elevated Cobra
Duration: 30 seconds each

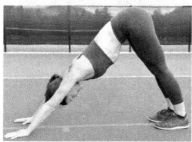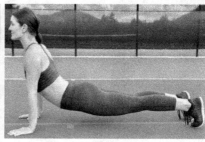

Drop down on your hands and knees with your hands under your shoulders and knees under your hips. Pike your hips up and pull them up and back toward your heels. Also pull your chest toward your knees. Try to straighten out your legs as much as you can without rounding your back. Next, let your hips and legs drop down toward the ground while letting your shoulder blades fall and back away from your ears. Tighten your thighs. These two exercises prepare your spine for flexion (bending forward) and extension (bending back) which are common and necessary motions for tennis.

SPIDERMANS
Repetitions: 5 each leg

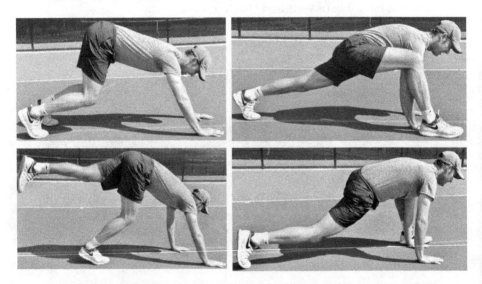

This is the dynamic portion of your warm-up. Start with your hands on the ground and your feet straight ahead with your hips up and knees bent. Step forward with one leg until your foot is right next to, and on the outside of, your hand. Make sure the foot is straight. Next, shift all your weight onto that front foot and bring the opposite leg into the air. Walk your hands forward several feet, and then step up with your back leg, placing your foot next to your hand. This dynamic movement lengthens your glutes and hip flexors and prepares your spine and both hips for bending, rotating and proper weight transfer.

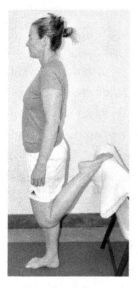

STANDING QUAD STRETCH
Duration: 1 minute

Place your foot behind you on a chair or on the net if you're on the court. You can also hold your own foot if needed. Keep your knees level, which you can see if you look down at your knees to notice if one knee is in front of the other. Tuck your hips under to increase the stretch on your thigh. This exercise is restoring full motion to your hip joint, which you'll need when playing. It's also preparing each hip to bear load properly.

Post-Tennis Cool-Down

The post-tennis routine is equally important. Tennis is an imbalanced sport, as you've already discovered. No matter how balanced and functional you are going in, I guarantee you'll be somewhat imbalanced coming out.

This routine will take seven to ten minutes and is designed to bring your body back to neutral by taking out all the twists and turns brought on by a mostly unilateral activity. It will also provide a mental and physical cooldown, and help you recover much faster overall so you're ready for the next day of hard-court (or clay court) fun.

Again, do these in order. If any of the exercises are painful or don't feel good, then skip it and go to the next one. At the end of the day what matters is what works for *you*.

COUNTER STRETCH
Duration: 1 minute

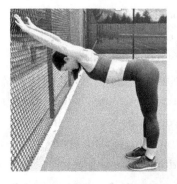

Place your hands on a fence or wall about chest height. Walk your legs back and bend at the waist as far as you can go keeping your hands on the wall and without sliding them down. Your ankles should be directly under your hips, your thighs should be engaged with your knees locked out and your feet should be six inches apart and pointing straight ahead. Lock out your elbows, but don't tug too much on your shoulders. You should feel no more than a light stretch or nothing at all in your arms and shoulders. Try to roll a slight arch in your low back, which will increase the stretch in the backs of your legs.

HIP CROSSOVER STRETCH
Duration: 1 minute each side

See instructions earlier in the chapter under the pre-tennis routine.

CATS AND DOGS
Repetitions: 10 cats and 10 dogs

See instructions earlier in the chapter under the pre-tennis routine.

DOWNWARD DOG
Duration: 1 minute

Use the same instructions as the downward dog in the pre-tennis routine, only without the elevated cobra to follow.

STATIC BACK PULLOVERS
Repetitions: 30

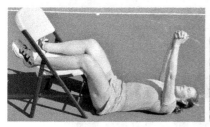 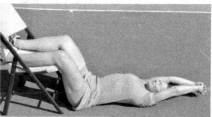

In the static back position (knees on a chair with hips and knees at 90 degrees), interlace your fingers together, keep your palms together, and straighten out your arms to lock your elbows. Pull your hands straight up overhead as far as you can go without bending your elbows. This exercise restores symmetry to your shoulders and back muscles, which also helps in balancing out your hips.

As you may have noticed, both routines are similar. They should be, considering they're both designed to restore balance to your muscles and joints. The only difference is the pre-routine is also meant to warm you up. Doing these exercises every time before and after you play will make a tremendous difference to how you feel on and off the court, especially when playing big matches where there's already a lot of tension.

One last thing—enjoy yourself out there. It's always more fun to play when your body feels good!

CHAPTER 27

THE NEW AND BALANCED YOU

N ow that you've done the self-assessment, understand the concept of imbalance, and addressed any pains you have, you're ready for the tools that will make you a functionally dominating tennis phenom. If you have any pain we didn't cover in the individual chapters, or if your pain lingers, don't despair.

The exercises given here address the position and function of your entire body, and since the body is a unit, by changing one part you can affect every other part. In other words, realigning your shoulders helps to balance and realign your hips, knees, and ankles. The same is true from the bottom up as it is the top down.

The goal of this menu is to correct the most common imbalances evident in all tennis players, as well as the ones you discovered in the self-assessment. Get back in touch with your weight distribution in your hips and feet and be sure to take notice of how you feel overall before doing the exercises.

Remember, it's imperative you know where you started so you can evaluate how much you've improved over the coming days and weeks.

The three most common responses I hear from my clients after the exercises are "I feel straighter," "I feel more evenly balanced," and "I feel better!" As long as you're paying attention and you stay connected to your body, you can't help but notice a significant change.

I also encourage you to take new pictures of yourself after a week of doing your exercises daily. Take them again after three weeks. When you compare those pics to the original ones you took you will see a difference. You might see your head position has moved back over your shoulders, or there is less rounding of your shoulders or your upper back, or your hips have come back over your ankles, or there is more curve in your lower back, or your feet are pointing straighter without thinking about it, or you just look better overall.

You might notice other differences on the tennis court. For example, you might feel more evenly balanced, you may notice that you're getting to balls you didn't get to before, or that you can serve bigger or more consistently, or that you're turning easier on your forehand and staying down better on your backhand. And much more.

I mentioned my own discoveries after starting the exercises—my back pain and ankle sprains disappeared. Plus, I was more balanced on the court, and felt better moving in general.

Here are the five most common postural imbalances in almost all tennis players:

1. One shoulder sits lower than the other.
2. One hip is rotated or sits higher than the other.
3. One foot turns out more than the other.
4. One shoulder is rounded forward more than the other.
5. There is an imbalanced weight distribution between the right and left foot (and hip).

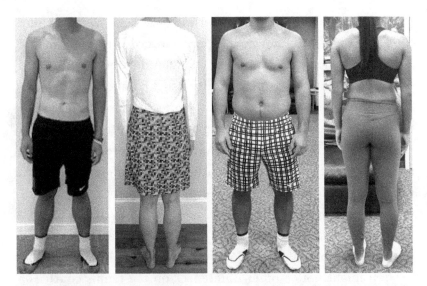

Figures 27.1-27.4 These are all very real, competitive tennis players. Notice the difference in shoulder level, one elevated and/or rotated forward hip, one hand in front of the other, one foot in front of the other, and the difference in weight distribution between right and left sides.

Of course, these postural deviations reflect common muscular imbalances that you can easily see or feel. For example:

- One calf muscle is usually larger than the other.
- One forearm is much bigger (obviously).
- Your back muscles on one side are more developed or overly engaged.
- The muscles that surround your hips are tighter on one side.
- Your oblique muscles (abs on the side) are tighter on one side.

You may have discovered many, or all, of these postural and muscular imbalances in yourself as you did the self-assessment. Every tennis player, and most athletes of all sports, have at least three of the postural imbalances listed above and most have four or five. You may have also found other deviations not listed above, like a forward head, hips swayed forward of your ankles and shoulders, or a rounded upper back.

These imbalances indicate how well your joints and muscles are functioning. They're also reflections of where your body is vulnerable to breaking down and more prone to injury and pain.

The good news is, whatever your twists, turns and postural imperfections, they will be addressed by this *Totally Balanced Tennis* routine. It's designed to tackle all of these imbalances from top to bottom, right to left and front to back. In case you need any further motivation, the potential short- and long-term benefits will be numerous, including:

- Injury prevention
- Faster injury recovery
- Restoring function, flexibility and motion to all your muscles and joints
- Feeling more balanced on and off the court
- Better movement
- Increased longevity in the sport
- More efficient strokes
- Increased energy
- Playing better tennis!

Before you dive in, there are a few tips to help you get the most out of the exercises:

Always do the exercises in the order listed.

The order matters because they're sequenced in a specific way that addresses the common muscular compensations followed by common root muscular and joint dysfunctions. The end goal is to leave your body connected and balanced with your joints in their neutrally aligned positions.

Pay strict attention to the form of each exercise.

Some of the exercises might be familiar to you, having done them in yoga, physical therapy, or somewhere else; some will be new. The key is how they're applied uniquely and specifically to you and to your particular imbalances. They're not chosen at random, and the particular form in which the exercise is done may be completely different than what you're used to. In that regard, the form is very important, and the specifics will be described with each one as you go along.

Hold each exercise for the fully recommended time.

Some exercises are counted by repetitions and sets; others are based on time. You want to hold the exercises for their fully allotted time because you'll notice some muscles begin to relax and others kick in. These are both signs the compensating muscles are letting go and the correct ones are waking up. You can hold an exercise longer than the prescribed time if you feel things releasing and you need longer; otherwise, set your timer and settle in.

Skip any exercise and go to the next one if it causes pain or discomfort beyond a normal stretch.

Always pay attention to your body and your instincts, and don't be afraid to skip anything that doesn't feel right. You can always come back to it later, and it might feel very different as your body changes.

Do the routine once a day for as many days a week as you can.

You can do the exercises every day seven days a week, or you can do them two to three days a week. The key is to find what works best for you. The more you do them, the more you'll benefit, but you have to balance your time with your instincts about your body and your goals.

This routine will take you forty-five minutes to start because you'll be reading the directions, watching the videos for form and taking your time. Once you get it down after about a week the routine will take you about twenty to twenty-five minutes. That's not much considering the ensuing benefit, and you'll really come to enjoy the routine because of how good you'll feel when you're done.

I recommend doing these exercises all at once, but you could break the routine up in two parts if you're stressed for time. If that's the case, you'd do the first six exercises ending with the static extension in the morning or on one day, then do the others later in the day or even the next day starting with the foot circles and point flexes.

In addition to the pictures and instructions here, you can watch the videos of these exercises at www.egoscue.com/agelesstennis.

The Totally Balanced Tennis Routine:

STANDING WINDMILL
Repetitions: 5 each direction in each position

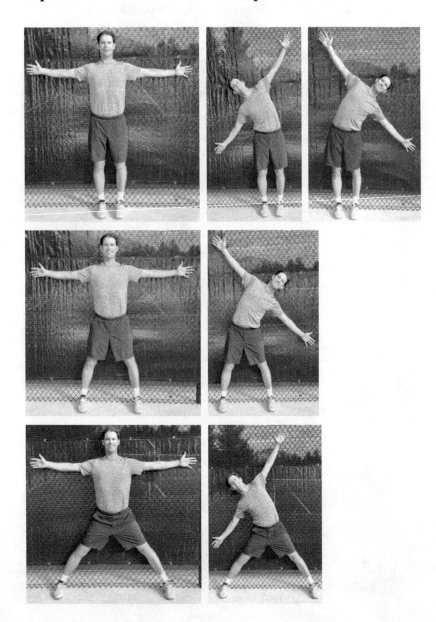

Start with your heels, hips, head, elbows and hands on a wall with your feet hip-width apart and pointing straight ahead. Your elbows should be locked straight out from your shoulders and your fingers spread. Keeping your thighs tight and your hips still (don't let them shift to the side), bend laterally to one side and then to the other as far as possible. Keep both heels down on the ground and imagine your arms are incapable of moving independent of your upper body. In other words, your arms go along for the ride, but don't drop them or raise them purposely. Go back and forth keeping your shoulders, backs of your hands, and head on the wall. After five reps to each side repeat, but widen your legs just short of as wide as you can. The final position is the same as the first, making it four positions total because you're starting and ending with your feet hip-width apart for a total of twenty repetitions (going from one side to the other is one repetition).

STATIC BACK ARM GLIDES
Repetitions: 30

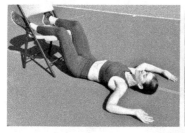 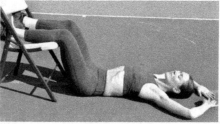

In the static back position (knees on a chair or couch with a 90-degree angle at the hips and knees) bend your elbows and let the backs of your hands fall toward the ground. Keeping your elbows, wrists and fingers on the ground and your elbows bent, slide your hands up above your head until they touch. Try not to arch your back off the ground as you raise your arms up. If you can't get your arms in this position or can't slide your hands over your head, then replace this exercise with the Kneeling Modified Counter Stretch in Chapter 21 page 142 in the section under swayed hips.

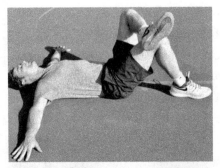

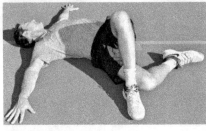

HIP CROSSOVER STRETCH
Duration: 1 minute each side

Lie on your back with your arms straight out from your shoulders, palms down, knees bent and feet on the ground. Cross your left ankle over your right knee and drop your right knee down to the right until the outside of your right leg and the bottom of your left foot are touching the ground. Press your left knee away from you with your leg muscles (not your hands), and turn your head to your left. Remember to keep your shoulders and palms flat on the ground and your elbows locked.

CATS AND DOGS
Repetitions: 10 cats and 10 dogs

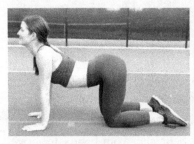
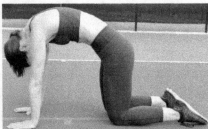

Go on your hands and knees with your hands directly under your shoulders and your knees directly under your hips. Let your back drop and your shoulder blades come together, but initiate the movement from your hips, not your spine. Look up as your back drops. Reverse directions by using your hips to begin to round your back up toward the sky and drop your head.

STATIC EXTENSION POSITION
Duration: 2 minutes

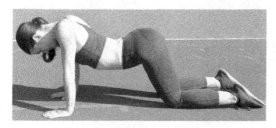

While on your hands and knees walk your hands forward until your hips are four to six inches in front of your knees. Keep your hands directly under your shoulders and let your shoulder blades drop together while you allow your chest to drop toward the ground. Keep your elbows straight and relax your chin down toward your chest. DO NOT MOVE YOUR HIPS TOO FAR FORWARD. If you feel you're in a modified push-up or your hips have dropped below your shoulders, you've probably gone too far.

FOOT CIRCLES POINT FLEXES
Repetitions: 40 circles each way and 40 point/flexes

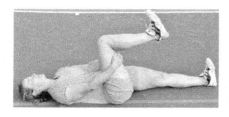

Begin by lying on your back and interlacing your hands under one knee while straightening out the opposite leg on the ground. Keep your shoulders relaxed down and back and the foot of the straight leg pointed toward the sky. Circle the foot of your bent knee one direction forty times, making as full a circle as you can, then switch directions. Once the circles are complete, point and flex your foot back and forth.

TRIANGLE
Duration: 1 minute

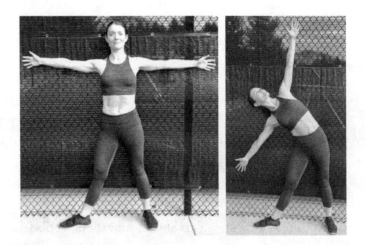

Stand against a wall with one heel, both hips, your upper back, head, and the backs of your hands on the wall with your arms straight out. Turn the other foot parallel to the wall, move it six inches away from the wall and place it outside of hip-width apart. Shift your weight onto the leg with the heel against the wall and bend laterally toward the turned-out foot. Tighten your thighs to lock out your knees, keep your shoulders, hips, and head on the wall and look up at your hands. Hold one minute, then switch sides.

CATS AND DOGS (AGAIN)

You do this exercise again to balance out your hip and spinal muscles after a rotation like the triangle.

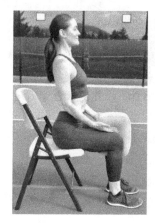

SITTING KNEE PILLOW SQUEEZES
Repetitions: 60

Sit toward the middle of a chair with your ankles directly under your knees and your hips rolled forward to create an arch in your low back. Place a pillow from your bed or couch (or a yoga block will do) and squeeze and release. Keep your feet straight and slightly less than hip-width apart. This exercise will remind your ankles, knees and hips to work together again and to bear balanced weight.

DOWNWARD DOG
Duration: 1 minute

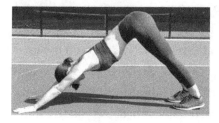

Drop on your hands and knees with your hands under your shoulders and knees under your hips. Pike your hips up and pull them up and back toward your heels. Pull your chest toward your knees to flatten out your back as much as you can. Keep your feet six inches apart and pointing straight ahead. If you can't do this without rounding your back, then bend your knees and flatten out your back (pull your chest toward your knees) with your knees bent.

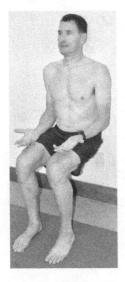

AIRBENCH
Duration: 2 minutes

Stand against the wall and walk your feet out as you slide your hips down the wall to just above 90 degrees. Press your low back flat into the wall and keep your feet pointing straight ahead. Your ankles should be slightly forward or directly under your knees and about six inches apart. You should be able to see your toes as you look down.

Congratulations! Now that you've completed the exercises, test your balance right to left and front to back. Walk around to notice how you feel and take note of what's changed. These exercises will get easier and your posture will continue to improve the more you do them. I advise doing *only* this functional routine specifically geared to your imbalances after you're out of pain from any individual pain menu.

If you're doing a lot of other activities, like Pilates, yoga, weight training, or any other exercise other than running, walking, or tennis, then I suggest that you stop for now. It matters because you're adding all those other exercises in the mix and it might be hard to distinguish what's doing what.

You need to act like a scientist and control as many variables as you can in order to accurately assess the results. You can definitely return to those other activities once you know how these exercises are changing you. In fact, all other forms of exercise and activity will feel very different in a good way, and you will get much more out of them once you're more balanced.

The goal here is to begin to teach you to be your own guide, feel your body, see and feel the impact of the exercises, and trust your instincts. Notice I use the word *feel* often. Feeling how all these exercises impact you is imperative, as opposed to just doing them and trusting they will help. I recognize that's challenging for some people because some are more kinesthetic than others.

If you're not one of those kinesthetic types, that's okay. Doing the self-assessment and diving into the exercises will give you a chance to practice being present and aware of your body. The pictures you take will also allow you to see the results, not just feel them, which will help validate their effectiveness.

In time, you'll begin to really connect with your body in a way you never had before, and you'll learn to trust your instincts, and your body's messages even more.

How long will it take to restore posture and function?

Many of you will see and feel a difference on and off the court after just one session. Postural change can happen immediately. You might notice other changes in your balance and symmetry occur gradually over several weeks. Functional change will follow the postural and positional change, and your nervous system will integrate it for good within several weeks or months.

Everyone, and I mean every single person reading this book, will change as long as you put in the time and effort, and you *maintain your awareness*. Staying connected to yourself and your body through these exercises will benefit you greatly.

Some people are skeptical that such simple exercises can be so effective in eliminating pain or in producing significant change. They can and they will, but don't just take my word for it. Try them and discover for yourself the change they can produce. Keep in mind, there is no downside to beginning the exercises, but there is a downside to never starting or to waiting too long.

This is your moment. This is your opportunity to change your body, and the course of your tennis career along with it.

Dive in, embrace the process of change, and reap the rewards that only a functional and balanced body can provide!

CHAPTER 28

TOTAL FUNCTIONAL STRENGTH

Functional strength is the harmonious marriage of full-joint mobility and joint stability with muscle endurance and power. Functional strength is required to hit a tennis ball, lunge for a backhand, jump for an overhead, and sprint for a drop shot, optimally without inducing injury. We want that strength.

The goal with functional strength training is to develop it, then enhance that muscle endurance and power to last through a match, or over several matches if in a tournament.

I would define dysfunctional strength as overly developed gym muscles that get in the way of any of the activities or put your body at risk of muscle imbalance and injury.

We get functional strength by training muscles and joints in all ranges of motion while enhancing stability. We get dysfunctional strength by strengthening some muscles more than others, and by not strengthening muscles and joints through their full range of motion.

I recently had a very well-known pro football player walk up to me during one of the team's strength workouts. He began to question his weight routines because he realized that although he was getting stronger, his body was feeling worse. His knees hurt, his neck was locked up, and it was still painful to run. His very words were "I'm done training like this. I'm all yours."

I took him out on the field, and we did forty-five minutes of what I consider functional strength training. Halfway through he said, "I haven't felt this worked over my whole body in a long time, and I can't remember the last time I felt this good."

This player is a veteran and relies on speed and power for his position. When we started, the lunge position irritated his painful knees. By the time we finished, not only could he lunge without any pain, but he could stay down in his stance (imperative for producing power), and sprinting felt free and easy.

A good functional strength workout should leave you feeling better than when you started—not worse. You might be tired, but it should be a good tired, and there should be very few, if any, lasting effects in the form of soreness. The best strength routines also target all your muscle groups and make them work together as a unit because muscles never work in isolation, especially during sports.

What you're really training in any strength routine is your nervous system, not the muscles. Your nervous system responds to the stimulus of the workout through the principle of adaptation. The adaptation in this case is an increase in muscle size and endurance, and your brain ingrains the pattern of movement to make that movement easier and more efficient the next time.

So, if you're considering an exercise at the gym, ask yourself if that's the pattern you want your nervous system to remember.

You can keep pounding the weights if you choose, but you should never do it to the detriment of form or function, and you should always mix it up. Alternatively, or additionally, you can follow the functional strength training menus I've created for you here, which hit all the muscles and joints. They're designed to take your body through a full range of motion, function, and strength. I guarantee you'll feel better, get stronger, and play better in the game of life, not to mention tennis.

You can pick one routine and do it for a week or a month, or you can do three different routines in a week if you feel like pushing yourself. The exercises are in a specific order, so do them in the order they appear. At the end of each routine I've included two or three quick exercises to reset your body after the workout. The reset exercises will help counteract any soreness while restoring your body back to neutral, and they will also help you recover.

I suggest only doing two to three strength workouts per week depending on how much tennis you're playing. If you're playing four to five times per week, then you might only want to do a strength routine twice per week. It's normal to be sore the first few times after doing these, but the muscle soreness will go away within a few days.

As usual, listen and pay attention to your body. Take a break when you're tired, and back off if you need to. It's always better to underdo it, rather than to overdo it.

Functional Tennis Strength #1

ABDOMINAL CRUNCHES
Repetitions: 100

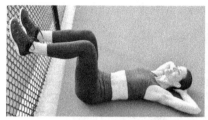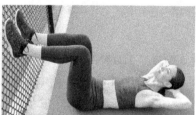

Rest your feet on a wall with your knees and hips bent at 90 degrees. Interlace your fingers together and pull your elbows back toward the ground. Keeping your elbows back and your hips on the ground, raise your upper body straight up about six to eight inches off the ground. It's important you keep your head and elbows back rather than pull both forward. It helps to look behind you or straight up at the sky as you come up.

BEARCRAWLS—FORWARD, SIDEWAYS, BACKWARD
Repetitions: 20 each direction

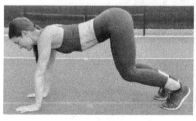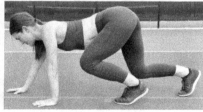

Start on all fours with your knees bent and hips in the air and equal weight between your hands and feet. Walk forward using your hands and feet at the same time so the weight stays equal in both. It's similar to crawling like you did when you were a kid, only this time your knees are in the air. Make sure as you crawl you keep your knees and feet tracking straight ahead rather than bringing your knees out to the sides. Try to keep your hips as still as possible as you crawl rather than let them sway side to side. Bearcrawl forward twenty times, sideways twenty times each direction and backward twenty times.

CIRCLE LUNGES
Repetitions: 4 to 6 complete circles

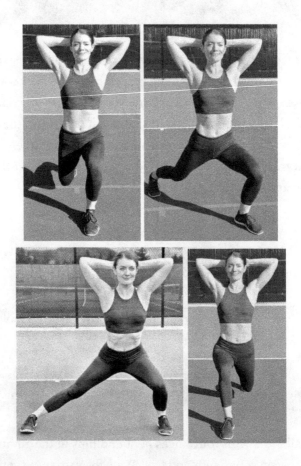

As the name implies you do a set of lunges in a complete circle. Start with your hands behind your head, fingers interlaced and your elbows pulled back. Step forward into a lunge position, keeping your foot straight and making sure your knee tracks straight ahead with your foot rather than collapsing in. Take a big step forward, then sink your hips toward the ground until your back knee almost touches the court, then step your feet back together. Next, lunge diagonally to 45 degrees, then straight out to the side, keeping your foot straight, and finally step directly behind you into a lunge and drop your hips down. Then switch legs and repeat. After completing a half circle with both legs that's one complete circle. Your goal is to do four to six complete circles. When those get easy add some weights to your hands or hold a medicine ball straight overhead.

TABLE SEQUENCE
Repetitions: 10 each position

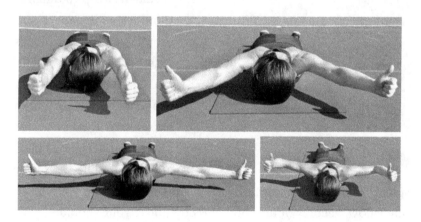

This exercise will wake up your shoulders as well as the muscles of your mid and upper back. Start face-down with your forehead on the ground and your feet pigeon-toed (toes touching, heels dropped out). Bring your arms straight out in front of you, make a fist with your thumbs up toward the sky, lock out your elbows and raise your hands and arms off the floor as high as you can. Hold for one to two seconds, then repeat ten times. Keep your head down as you raise your arms up! Repeat with your arms at 45 degrees, then again at 90 degrees. For the final position, bend your elbows to 90 degrees keeping your thumbs pointing straight up toward the sky, and lift your hands and elbows as high as you can. When this sequence gets easy you can hold one-to-three-pound weights in your hands. Good luck!

CORE ABS—4 POSITIONS
Duration: 1 minute each position

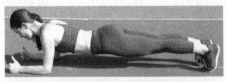
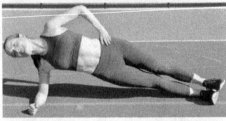
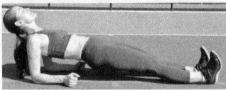

Drop down to your elbows and straighten your legs out behind you. Lift your body off the ground until your hips are level with your shoulders. Keep your hands shoulder-width apart and drop your shoulder blades together until they touch. Make sure your hips don't drop. Tighten your thigh muscles to lock out your knees, and keep your head and neck in line with your spine. For the second position, roll to your side and hold yourself on one elbow, keeping your elbow directly under your shoulder, your thumb up toward the sky, your thighs contracted and stacked on one another, and your feet flexed back. Finally, lie on your back with your elbows underneath you propping you up and directly under your shoulders. Keep your thighs contracted and feet flexed back toward your knees and lift your hips and upper body off the ground as high as you can. This sequence never gets old and takes time to get easy, but when it does just add more time.

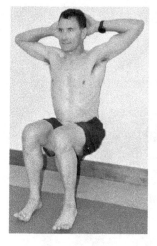

DECLINE AIRBENCH
Duration: 1 minute

Lean against a wall with your knees bent at 90 degrees. Make sure your ankles are slightly forward or directly under your knees and slide down so your hips are slightly below your knees. Press your low back into the wall, interlace your fingers behind your head and pull your elbows back to the wall. Lift your toes up off the ground and don't forget to smile. It's already difficult, but you can always increase the time to make it tougher.

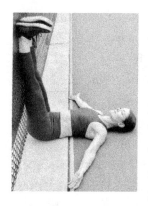

STATIC WALL
Duration: 4 minutes

This is the reset exercise to reset your body back to neutral. Lie on your back with your legs up a wall and your hips touching the wall. Tighten your thighs, flex your feet back, relax your upper body completely with your hands out to your sides and your palms up. Breathe in and out from your diaphragm, close your eyes and give yourself kudos for a job well done.

Funtional Tennis Strength Routine #2

STANDING ARM CIRCLES
Repetitions: 60 forward, palms down; 60 backward, palms up

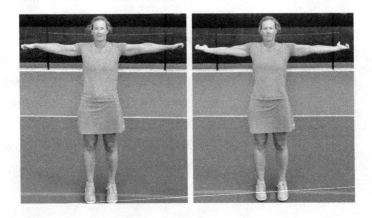

Stand with your feet straight, your arms straight out from your shoulders and your shoulder blades squeezed together. Think of pulling your shoulders down and back away from your ears. Make what we call a golfer's grip with your hands where you spread your fingers out and then curl the top knuckles tight into the palms of your hands. Keep your feet pointing straight ahead and about six to eight inches apart. Relax your stomach. With your thumbs pointing straight ahead make small circles at a medium pace in the direction of your thumb. To be clear, begin by circling up and in the direction of your thumb. Do sixty circles, then rotate your palms up, keeping the same grip, and do sixty circles backward.

Imagine doing circles around your own fist as a gauge of how big they should be.

WALKOUTS
Repetitions: 10, 9, 8, 7, 6, 5, 4, 3, 2, 1

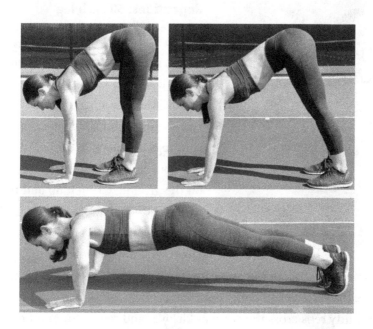

This exercise starts with you bending down like you're going to touch your toes. Your feet should be pointing straight ahead and six inches apart. From there walk your hands out into a push-up position keeping your hips level with your shoulders and your knees locked (do not let them bend). Do ten push-ups with your shoulder blades squeezed together the whole time and your thigh muscles contracted, then walk your hands back to your feet *without bending your knees.* Use your hips to help pull your body back to the starting position, then walk back out to the push-up position again, but this time do nine push-ups. Walk back to the starting position, then back out for eight push-ups . . . all the way to one.

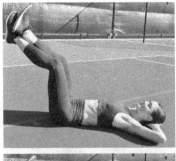

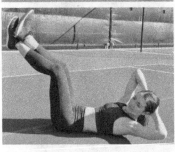

Free Crunches with Obliques
Repetitions: 50 each leg

Lie on your back with your legs in the air, your fingers interlaced behind your head and your elbows pulled back. Cross one ankle over the other and slightly bend your knees. Lower your legs down just a little until you feel your lower back barely raise up off the ground. Crunch up and twist to one side as you raise your body, but keep your elbows and head back. Drop back down and raise up again, this time twisting to the opposite side. Don't let your head or elbows come forward as you come up. Each crunch with a twist is one rep. After fifty reps cross the other ankle over and repeat for another set.

Supermans/Superwomans
Repetitions: 10 with 10-second hold

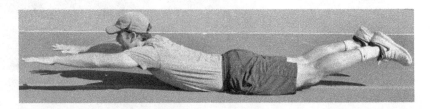

Lying on your stomach with your arms in front of you, raise your arms, head, upper body and legs as high as you can. Point your toes, look straight ahead and hold for ten seconds.

CATS AND DOGS
Repetitions: 20

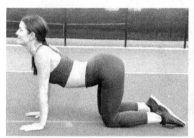 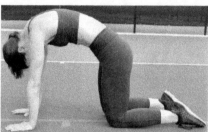

SIDE SQUAT WALKS WITH HANDS BEHIND HEAD
Repetitions: 15 to 20 each direction

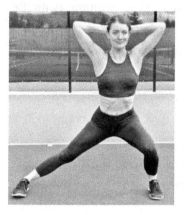

Begin in a squatting position with your feet pointed straight ahead, your fingers interlaced behind your head and your elbows pulled back. Drop your hips as low as you can, then take a big step out to the side keeping your foot straight when you land. Transfer your weight to that foot, bring the other back to the starting position and repeat. Keep your hips down the entire time, look straight ahead, and keep your elbows pulled back.

Double Leg Hops
Repetitions: 20

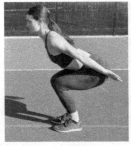 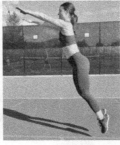 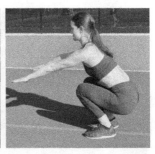

Bring your feet straight and hip-width apart. Drop your hips down low keeping your upper body as upright as possible. Jump evenly off both feet as high and far as you can. When you land, land evenly on both feet and let your hips sink back down before jumping again. Be as explosive as you can and pay close attention to your form. You MUST jump evenly off both feet and land evenly on both feet.

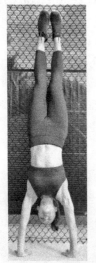

Handstand
Duration: 1 minute

You have two choices of how to do this exercise. You can face the wall, drop down on your hands and kick your legs up like the model in the picture, or you can start on your hands and knees facing away from the wall and walk your feet up the wall as far as you can while you walk your hands toward the wall. If you walk your feet up the wall you'll end up facing the wall rather than away from it like the model. Either way, lock out your elbows, straighten up your legs and get as close to the wall as you can. Your goal is one minute, but come out of the exercise before you get too tired. You don't want those arms to collapse!

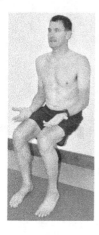

Airbench
Duration: 2 minutes

Lean against a wall, drop down to just above 90 degrees, walk your feet out so your ankles are directly under or just in front of your knees (you should be able to see you toes). Unlike the stud in the picture, wear shoes so your feet don't slip. Press your low back flat into the wall and hang out!

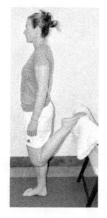

Standing Quad Stretch
Duration: 1 to 2 minutes

Place your foot behind you on a chair or on the net if you're on the court. You can also hold your own foot if needed. Keep your knees level, which you can check by looking down at your knees to observe if one is in front of the other. Tuck your hips under to increase the stretch on your thigh.

Static Back
Duration: 5 to 10 minutes

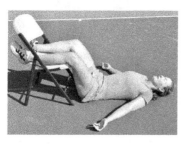

Ahhhhhh... Put your legs up on a chair with your hips nestled up to it as close as you can. Your goal is 90 degrees at the hips and knees. Relax your arms out to your sides with your palms up and breathe. You killed this workout and you earned a well-deserved rest as your back and hip muscles rebalance top to bottom and right to left.

Functional Tennis Strength #3—Appropriate for ANY Age and Athletic Ability

ARM CIRCLES

Repetitions: 50 palms down going forward and 50 palms up going back

See the picture and explanation earlier in this chapter.

3 POSITION TOE RAISES

Repetitions: 10 each position, repeat 3x

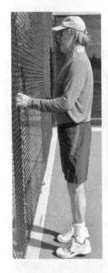 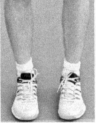 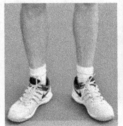 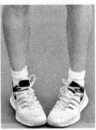

Stand upright with your feet straight and six inches apart, holding on to a doorway, fence or pole. Rise up on your toes as high as you can without leaning forward. The pole or fence helps you keep your hips back over your ankles rather than pitching forward as you come up on your toes. Your goal is to keep your upper body completely straight.

After ten toe raises turn your feet out to 45 degrees and repeat, then again with your toes touching and your heels apart. Keep your knees locked out, your thighs tight, and make sure as you come up you keep your weight on the insides of your feet rather than letting your feet roll to the outside.

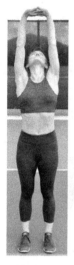

STANDING OVERHEAD EXTENSION
Duration: 1 minute

Stand with your feet straight and six inches apart. Interlace your fingers together and turn your palms away from you. Bring your hands straight up overhead while locking out your elbows. Pull back as far as you can and reach for the sky. Don't let your hips shift forward like you're in a backbend. Instead, keep your hips over your heels. Look up toward your hands, relax your stomach and hold.

PUSH-UPS
Repetitions: 25

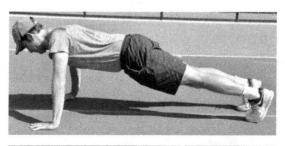

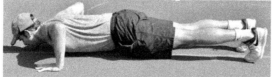

This is just like a traditional push-up, only your shoulder blades are squeezed together, your thigh muscles stay contracted to keep your legs completely straight and your hips stay level with your shoulders the entire time. Keep your arms wider than shoulder width and try to go as low as you can.

ABDOMINAL CRUNCHES
Repetitions: 50

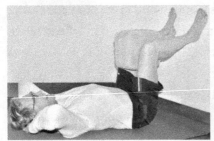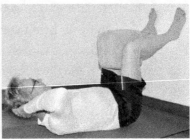

Your hips and knees are at 90 degrees with a pillow between your knees. Make sure your feet are pointing straight ahead and are less than hip-width apart. Keep 70 percent pressure on the pillow as you bring your upper body straight up off the ground keeping your head and your elbows pulled back.

ACTIVE BRIDGES
Repetitions: 25

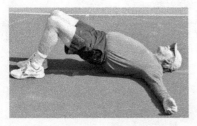 Lie on your back with your knees bent and feet on the ground pointing straight ahead. Rest your arms out to the sides. Push your hips up as high as they can go, then bring them back down. Repeat.

CATS AND DOGS
Repetitions: 20

You know the drill. Go slowly and initiate all motion with your hips.

SIT-TO-STANDS
Repetitions: 15-20

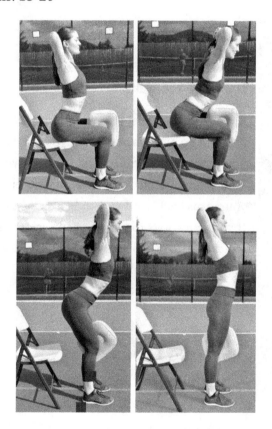

Sit on a bench or in the middle of a chair with a pillow between your knees, your ankles directly under your knees, your feet straight, and your hips and knees at 90 degrees. Interlace your fingers behind your head and pull your elbows back. Create an arch in your low back by rolling your hips forward. Stand up from that position trying not to lean forward as much as possible and without sliding your feet back. I know; it's not as easy as it sounds. But that's the challenge. Keep constant pressure on the pillow as you come up; then sit back down in the same way you got up—your elbows are pulled back, there's an arch in your back and you're looking straight ahead. Once again, don't slide your feet back to stand up (that's cheating). Keep your knees at 90 degrees and your ankles directly under your knees not behind them.

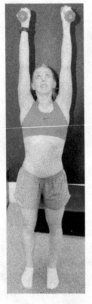

STATIC DUMBELL PRESS
Duration: 1 minute

Stand with your feet straight about fist-width apart. Holding no more than two to five pounds, straighten up your arms overhead and lock out your elbows. Your palms should be facing each other as you pull your arms back overhead and look up at your hands. If your neck gets too tired, then look straight ahead instead of up. Keep your hips back over your ankles and relax your stomach.

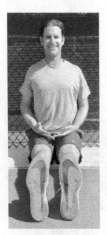

SITTING FLOOR
Duration: 3 minutes

Sit down on the ground with your back against a wall and your legs straight out in front of you. Bring your feet about four to six inches apart and point your feet straight up toward the sky. Flex your thigh muscles and push your knees straight down into the floor. Pull back from the outsides of your feet to make sure they're flat rather than angled and squeeze your shoulder blades down and back with as much force as you can muster and hold.

CATS AND DOGS

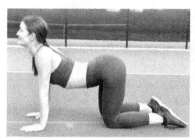 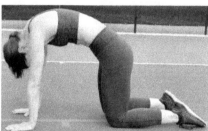

Go on your hands and knees with your hands directly under your shoulders and your knees directly under your hips. Let your back drop and your shoulder blades come together, but initiate the movement from your hips, not your spine. Look up as your back drops. Reverse directions by using your hips to begin to round your back up toward the sky and drop your head.

FREE SQUAT
Duration 30 seconds to 1 minute

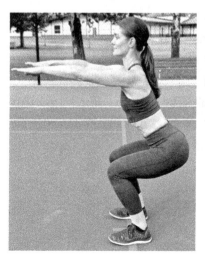

With both feet straight and hip-width apart squat down by dropping your hips to just above 90 degrees. Keep an arch in your low back, look straight ahead and keep your upper body up (try not to lean forward). This exercise resets the trunk over the hips and forces the body to evenly weight both sides.

CHAPTER 29

HYDRATION—
IT'S TIME TO DRINK

I'm sure by this point you've heard enough about the importance of hydration to last a lifetime, but I'm going to be your imaginary, overly concerned mother for a second in order to drive home the message.

I'll start with a quick anecdote.

I was playing in the first round of a big open tournament in California where I had high expectations. I had been training hard and playing well leading up to it, having notched some big wins and breakthroughs just a few weeks before. I started out serving big, feeling great, and playing even better. I went up 5-2 in the first set when the wheels started coming off.

All at once I began to get a small headache, felt overheated, lost all my energy, and began to feel slightly nauseous. I lost eight straight games before pulling it together, only to strain a hamstring muscle just as I began to mount a comeback up breakpoint at 2-4.

What happened? Dehydration that led to early symptoms of heat stroke and a slight injury. I had flown in from the East Coast the afternoon before (not ideal preparation), jumped on the court to hit, and within ten minutes my calf cramped. I knew I was dehydrated, but I figured I would be fine by the next day in time for my match at 11:30. I wasn't. It was a good lesson in the value of drinking enough.

Every one of the cells that make up every bone, muscle, joint, tendon, and nervous tissue in our bodies contains anywhere from 30 percent to 90 percent water. Your muscles, heart, brain and kidneys are about 75 percent water (give or take depending on your size, muscle mass). Your blood is just under 80 percent water. Even your bones are composed of about 33 percent water. All this water indicates that you are basically one very large, moving, tennis playing, highly intelligent, kickass water molecule.

Of the many roles water plays, one of them is to function as a cushion for our joints and spines. The spinal discs, which sit in between the vertebrae, act as cushions and shock absorbers and are also comprised of about 80 percent water.

Any kind of dehydration will impede their ability to function optimally, but the more dried out they get, the more brittle they become, and the less cushion they're able to provide. Brittle intervertebral discs are also more vulnerable to breaking much like a cracker in too thick a dip. Once a disc breaks or ruptures it can impinge some major nerves in your spine that are much better left alone. Trust me when I say you don't want to get to that point because debilitating pain could be the least of your worries.

The same is true for joints in terms of dehydration. Water provides cushion and lubrication between every joint in the body. If you are dehydrated, so are your joints, and they can no longer provide the sufficient viscosity and glide they once did. Imagine not having enough oil in your car to provide lubrication to your engine; we all know how that ends. Similarly, a lack of water in your joints creates friction, irritation, pain, and eventually injury.

In terms of muscles, a dehydrated muscle can't transfer force as effectively, protect your joints, or move as efficiently. It will also tear more easily.

How can you tell if you're dehydrated? Loss of energy, feeling sleepy or fatigued, a decrease in performance, muscle or joint pain, and even hunger can all be signs of dehydration. If you can't focus on the court, if you aren't thinking clearly, or you feel like your coordination is slightly off, chances are you need to drink some water. You might also need to eat something to raise your blood sugar.

How much water is enough to keep you juicy? There are so many recommendations out there on how much to drink to stay hydrated: Drink eight-ounce glasses of water a day, drink ten glasses of fluid a day, drink half your body weight in ounces every day, and so forth.

I'm sure these are all great suggestions, and if you're not sure what to do, just pick one and see how it works for you. And no, the ice in your Scotch doesn't count as drinking water. Alcohol and caffeine tend to draw water away from your cells.

Personally, I recommend drinking a glass of water immediately upon waking up because after sleeping your body has been without water for eight to ten hours. You're dehydrated whether you know it or not. Drinking water upon waking will also kick-start your metabolism and lubricate all the things that need lubricating upon waking, like your throat and your digestive system.

In addition to that initial glass, drink whenever you feel thirsty, or have at least one glass of water every two hours, including one at night before you go to sleep. Yes, you might have to pee in the middle of the night, but you'll sleep better overall, and it will help combat that groggy feeling of "I need to hit the snooze button five times" when your alarm goes off.

On the court, I recommend hydrating between every changeover (duh), or if you're practicing, take a chug of water every five minutes. I know, it seems so obvious that I sound like the flight attendant telling you how to buckle your seatbelt. But I'd bet there's at least one person reading this right now who rarely drinks while playing. If that's you, cut the "I don't need it, I'm fine" crap and start hydrating.

In the meantime, there are several great books about water. I highly recommend "Your Body's Many Cries for Water" by the late Dr. Fereydoon Batmanghelidj.

So, are you feeling sufficiently motivated to start pounding the H2O? If not, let me add that in addition to the myriad of negative side effects of dehydration, if you're even a little dehydrated you simply cannot play your best tennis. It's not physically possible. So, drink up.

CHAPTER 30

TIPS FROM THE TOP

"Tips from the Top" was a phrase my dad used to use when he was coaching me as a junior player. He was a pro-hockey-player-turned-tennis-enthusiast at a late age, so he would pass on advice to me that he had heard or read from top coaches and pros, hence the catchy moniker.

We joke about it now, and the saying is still fondly and frequently recalled when he feels the need to impart his fatherly wisdom to his grateful son to this day. I use it now as homage to him and to pass on my own final tips and thoughts to you:

- The more functional you become, the more of your tennis potential you can fulfill.
- The body always operates as one big interconnected and interdependent unit, and it should be treated and trained as such.
- The quality of your movement and your strokes is dependent on the position, the stability, and the mobility of *all* your joints.
- The site of the pain is rarely the cause of the pain.
- Everything in your body is alive, which gives it an almost unlimited capacity to heal.

- Treat the position of your body, not just the condition. More often than not, the condition will take care of itself by fixing the root cause.
- Listen to your body; it will tell you everything you need to know.
- Pain is a message. Don't ignore it, and be careful when deadening it.
- The pain isn't due to the activity or sport; it's due to the body you bring to the sport.
- Straighten before you strengthen.
- Mobility and stability together beget strength, not the other way around.
- Core strength is about balanced muscles, not strong ones.
- Static stretching works to unravel the layers of muscle compensation and reprograms the central nervous system.
- Dynamic stretching and dynamic movement work better when you balance the body first.
- The more aligned and muscularly balanced you are, the better you'll feel and the better you'll play.
- Weightlifting can be helpful, but it can also be harmful, and often is. Pay attention to form and focus on balanced muscles, not just the ones that stand out in the mirror.
- Be patient. The difference you feel after doing the exercises can be immediate, but the process of total change takes time.
- The pre- and post-tennis menus are imperative to finding balance before and after you play.
- With some work and dedication, you can enjoy this sport throughout the long years of your life, not to mention becoming a functionally dominating tennis phenom!

Yoda's parting words to Luke were, "Pass on what you have learned." I hope I've done that to some meaningful and impactful degree, and I hope you will too. Your body, with its infinite and evolutionary wisdom, has always been, and will continue to be, your best teacher. It will relay everything you need to know about your health and what it needs to thrive. As long as you stay connected to it, and to yourself, you can't lose.

YOUR BRILLIANT INNER VOICE

had to learn how to be responsible for my health. Nobody told me that doctors don't always have all the answers, and when they didn't solve my chronic back pain, I felt powerless. After all, if they couldn't help me, who could? Me? What did I know about the body?

I have tremendous respect for the hard-working and wonderful doctors, physical therapists, and others of the allopathic world. They are the first experts I would go to if I broke a bone or if I was convinced that surgery was the best or only option. Indeed, they are often the first experts I refer my clients to when I suspect there's an underlying medical condition that the exercises I prescribe just can't treat.

Doctors are under a lot of pressure—too much pressure—from a culture that often expects them to have all the answers. They don't, and they were never supposed to. They have answers to specific questions, but not all the answers.

Personally, when it comes to chronic spine, muscle, or joint pain, I regard the current Western model of care as simply part of a larger wheel of potential healthcare choices. Obviously, depending on your needs and preferences, there's absolutely a time and a place for it, just as there's a time and a place for alternative routes such as acupuncture, Rolfing, Muscle Activation Technique, chiropractic care, energy healing, and many other modalities. The key to successful healing and treatment is understanding when and how to use each modality.

The truth is, your doctors, acupuncturist, chiropractor and other health practitioners are merely guides. We all have our advice for you, and although our intentions are pure, some of it will fit you like a tailor-made suit, and some of it will only weigh you down and sag like old underwear. Therefore, it's imperative you learn to become your own guide.

To that end, I encourage you to try many different healing paths so you can expand your network of health and wellness professionals and, thus, your options. At the end of the day, there are many ways to heal and many roads to health and happiness. What's most important is what works for you.

Of course, deciding on which road to follow and whose advice to take can be challenging, if not sometimes overwhelming.

These are the times to get in touch with the knower inside you, that grounded and wise part of you, the brilliant inner voice enabling you to make the best decision you can at the time. While that path you choose might not be perfect, it will eventually lead you to one that is.

Once you take control of your health by trusting your instincts, getting in touch with your body's internal messages, and acting on that information, you trigger your body's practically unlimited capacity to heal.

In the end there are two universal truths when it comes to your health: You are the expert on your body, and nobody heals you; you heal yourself.

FAQS

If I want better posture, should I pull my shoulders back consciously?

No. The exercises will strengthen your muscles and your posture, so you don't have to walk around thinking about it all day long. After all, I'm sure you have more important things to do than worry about whether or not you're standing up straight. What you can do consciously from time to time is stand on both feet rather than shift your hips off to one leg.

Should I consciously keep my stomach engaged and tight?

Definitely not. Your stomach should be relaxed and moving as you breathe. It should also be relaxed during the exercises. Your diaphragm is supposed to be allowed to expand and contract fully as you breathe, and it can't do that if you're holding your stomach in. There are myriad other issues that come with holding your stomach in, which range from emotional to physical, but for the sake of space on this page I'll just say, *breathe*!

Is it okay if I wear orthotics?

Yes and no. If you need orthotics to stay out of pain, then go for it. If you're wearing orthotics because someone told you to, I suggest you wean yourself off them as you strengthen the muscles of your feet and ankles via the exercises. The orthotics are trying to compensate for the weak and dysfunctional muscles of your feet and even your hips, so as you strengthen those muscles you hopefully won't need the orthotics. Also, orthotics will restrict the motion of your feet (like casts), and when you take them out your feet go back to doing what they've always done.

Do I have to do the exercises every day?

There's a saying, "Only brush the teeth you want to keep." Only strengthen the muscles you want to keep too. Our bodies are use-it-or-lose-it mechanisms. If you do the exercises every day, then you're a rock star. If you do the exercises three to five days a week, I'm sure you'll gain ground and make progress. If you do the exercises once a week, you're probably still doing yourself a favor, but it's hard to say to what extent.

I suggest you shoot for four to seven days a week in the beginning, and over time you'll figure out how many days a week works the best to maximize and maintain your gains.

Is it okay to take a break from the exercises sometimes?

Yes, yes, and yes. If you feel your body is overworked, then take a break. If any of the exercises are causing pain or soreness that isn't going away, then skip it or pick a new routine. Sometimes your body just needs to rest and do nothing, and that can be the absolute best healing and most loving thing you can do for yourself.

Do I need any equipment, and if so, where can I get it?

The exercises are designed to be done in your home or on the court with very little to no equipment except what you might have already in your house.

You can also go to your local *Egoscue* clinic for help if there's one in your city. You can find out at www.egoscue.com.

What if the pain doesn't go away?

There's never a downside to seeing a doctor if you haven't already seen one because at the very least you'll be armed with more information, and they're there to help. You can also seek out other help in the form of another health practitioner that has experience with your issue.

If you've seen docs and health practitioners galore and nothing has helped, including these exercises, then you might need something more specific to you, which you can get at an *Egoscue* clinic. I suggest making an appointment to be seen by a therapist either in the clinic or via Skype. Go to www.egoscue.com for more information or to make an appointment.

Do you see people individually for sessions?

I do, but if you don't live in San Francisco, I usually either work with you via Skype or online where I can talk to you, look at your pictures, and then create a routine specific to you. You can always email me at agelesstennis@gmail.com.

What do you think of band work, med ball training, Pilates, yoga, etc?

I love it all. The questions are what do you love to do, and how much variety are you getting? The more you vary your activities and your workouts, the better. I like yoga for the varied positions it offers, which can stimulate your body's need for motion in many different planes. However, in any activity if you're not paying attention to your body or your instincts, or if your ego is in the way, then you can hurt yourself.

Whatever activity you do, ask yourself how you feel after. If you feel great, then it was probably good for you. If you don't feel great, or you're in some pain, then it probably wasn't that good for you and you should consider taking a break or finding a different form of exercise.

RECOMMENDED RESOURCES

Here are some other resources I love and highly recommend on your journey to playing your best tennis, and to finding the best practices for your body, your mind, and your long-term health.

- *Pain Free* **by Pete Egoscue**
  This is a wonderful resource for anyone experiencing chronic muscle or joint pain and a great companion to this book.

- *The Best Tennis of Your Life* **by Jeff Greenwald**
  This is a fantastic book to hone your mental skills and to reach the next level in your game. He provides useful and easy tips to incorporate on and off the court that will make a huge impact on your results.

- *4-Hour Body* **by Tim Ferriss**
  This is a unique, interesting, informative and highly entertaining read. Even if you don't use any of the advice, I guarantee you'll learn something about your body and your health along the way.

- **www.egoscue.com**
  Head to this website If you're dealing wtih chronic musculoskeletal pain, want to learn more about Egoscue, become a therapist or make an appointment at a clinic near you.

- ***Your Body's Many Cries for Water* by Fereydoon Batmanghelidj**
  You'll be surprised at what you learn about hydration and you'll never pass on that extra glass of water again.

- ***Will You Still Love Me If I Don't Win?* by Christopher Andersonn**
  If we've covered the physical and mental aspects of the body with the other books, this one tackles the emotional side. Filled with helpful insights on what children experience in athletics and how to help them on their journey, this is a must read for all parents of aspiring athletes.

ACKNOWLEDGMENTS

This book was born of love. It combines my love of the body and postural therapy and my love of tennis. It embodies the love of all four of my parents, who always encouraged me to pursue my truth and follow my own path. It took Pete Egoscue and his love for helping people he's never met to help illuminate that path. If it wasn't for the love and support of my partner, Teresa, I may not have stuck with it. And finally, it took John Koehler and his fantastic team's love for their craft to bring this entire manuscript to life.

Thank you, all of you.

CPSIA information can be obtained
at www.ICGtesting.com
Printed in the USA
LVHW022257280920
667360LV00002B/360